Excessive Medical Spe

Facing the challenge

Excessive Medical Spending

Facing the challenge

Edited by

Norman J. Temple
Athabasca University

and

Andrew Thompson
University of Oregon (retired)

Radcliffe Publishing
Oxford • Seattle

Radcliffe Publishing Ltd
18 Marcham Road
Abingdon
Oxon OX14 1AA
United Kingdom

www.radcliffe-oxford.com
Electronic catalogue and worldwide online ordering facility.

British Library Cataloguing in Publication Data

A catalogue record for this book is available from the British Library.

ISBN-10   1 84619 168 8
ISBN-13   978 1 84619 168 8

Typeset by Advance Typesetting Ltd, Oxford, UK
Printed and bound by Biddles Ltd, King's Lynn, Norfolk, UK

To Michael and Gillian
– Norman

To my wife, Marie-Anne, for putting up with me
– Andrew

Contents

Foreword ix

Author addresses xii

Introduction xiv

1 The cost of medical care: how much is too much? 1
Andrew Thompson and Norman J. Temple

2 The nuts and bolts of medical research 9
Norman J. Temple and Andrew Thompson

3 Conflict of interest: a major problem in medical research 20
Joy Fraser

4 Drug regulation: two paradigms in conflict 36
Joel Lexchin

5 The marketing of drugs: how drug companies manipulate the
prescribing habits of doctors 53
Audrey Balay-Karperien, Norman J. Temple, and Joel Lexchin

6 Pricing pharmaceutical drugs in the USA 63
Donald W. Light

7 Potential savings from therapeutic substitution of 10 of Canada's
most dispensed prescription drugs 80
Alan Cassels and Joel Lexchin

8 Statins: is the net being thrown too wide? 93
Andrew Thompson and Norman J. Temple

9 Modern Western medicine: lots of bucks – where's the bang? 101
Norman J. Temple and Joy Fraser

10 Genetics, genomic medicine, and achieving better population health:
a flawed strategy? 110
Patricia A. Baird and Norman J. Temple

11 Issues in screening for cancer 112
Luc Bonneux

12 The Canadian National Breast Screening Study: science meets
controversy 121
Cornelia J. Baines

13 Screening for breast cancer: benefits versus costs 125
Andrew Thompson and Norman J. Temple

14 Screening for cervical cancer by Pap tests 131
Andrew Thompson and Norman J. Temple

15 Paying for what works: the Reference Drug Program as a model
for rational policy-making 139
Alan Cassels and Norman J. Temple

16 Disease prevention: the neglected alternative 152
Norman J. Temple

17 Promoting the health of the medical profession: environmentalism
and commercialism in medical education 166
Iahn Gonsenhauser, Danny George, and Peter J. Whitehouse

18 A proposed new grand strategy: an integrated health system for
the 21st century 177
Norman J. Temple and Andrew Thompson

Index 187

Foreword

Every industrialized society in the world is aging rapidly. With life expectancies at all-time highs and birth rates near all-time lows, the Baby Boom generation is closing in on retirement – a time when healthcare needs escalate rapidly – with relatively fewer young people around to pay the bills. While most discussions about the fiscal problems caused by aging societies have focused on pensions and income security, the more serious landmine in the road ahead is healthcare finance, which will be in full-blown crisis sometime early in the next decade. That's why this book, *Excessive Medical Spending: Facing the Challenge*, is timely. Until we learn to talk openly and honestly about what constitutes good health, good healthcare, and the best and most cost-effective way of achieving both, we will never have an affordable healthcare system.

The current practice of medicine, which is dominated by pharmaceutical and medical device companies, hospital chains, physicians' guilds, and, in the case of the USA, large insurers, is designed to avoid asking such questions. Even countries with single-payer national healthcare systems have been stymied in their attempts to curb the influence of the special interests. The result is that in most industrialized countries healthcare spending is growing two or three times faster than the rest of the economy. The USA is leading the charge into healthcare bankruptcy by spending nearly 15% of its gross domestic product on health, a level nearly 50% greater than any other nation. Formerly great industrial powerhouses like General Motors and Ford are now threatened by economic collapse because of their escalating healthcare costs.

So the time has come to ask some hard questions about what we are getting for our large and growing investment in health. Yes, we are living longer, but are medical interventions the reason? To an extent they are, but are they adding as much to our quality of life as they are to its duration? Are there some healthcare interventions that are simply not worth the price? And are there better ways of addressing underlying healthcare problems that not only extend life, but do so at lower cost and with better outcomes in terms of our ability to enjoy our extra months and years?

In order to answer such questions, we need a new language for talking about how we spend our healthcare dollars. Take heart disease, for example. Though it remains a leading killer in virtually every wealthy nation, death rates from cardiovascular disease have been edging down in recent decades. What accounts for the improvement? Can it be attributed to advances in diagnostics, drug therapy, and implantable devices such as stents and defibrillators? Or has it largely been due to public health campaigns to combat smoking, poor diets, and lack of exercise? And now that we are facing an alarming situation where some of those gains may be reversed because of the obesity epidemic, what is the best strategy for preserving and extending our gains against this feared disease?

As the studies here show, physicians seeking guidance for their treatment decisions will not get an objective review of the evidence when they go to the medical literature or read clinical practice guidelines. Drug companies and device manufacturers have financed study after study showing that their proprietary intervention lowers the risk of disease by some percentage, usually reported as relative risk. Headlines written from such studies shout that taking the pill will reduce your chance of suffering a heart attack by 30%! What they fail to tell you is that 50 or 100 people need to take the pill before one gets the benefit.

One recent study among people who had already suffered a heart attack showed that the most expensive intervention – a brand name statin at high doses that can cost upwards of $1000 a year – insignificantly reduced further heart disease and lowered cardiovascular mortality not at all when compared to a low-dose statin soon to go generic. Yet the accompanying editorial touted the high-dose approach.[1] What that study and so many others like it failed to do was compare either drug therapy approach to alternatives like lifestyle intervention, even though switching to a Mediterranean-style diet could cut a patient's risk of a second heart attack in half.[2] Unfortunately, few regulatory bodies around the world require comparison studies when approving new medical interventions.

The USA is among the worst in this regard. As one high official at the Food and Drug Administration once explained it, drug companies do not have to prove the fifth or sixth ACE inhibitor is better than the others at lowering blood pressure; it need only prove that it is better than nothing.[3] The idea that regulators might require that ACE inhibitors be compared to other classes of blood pressure medications (as was done in the ALLHAT trial, which showed that generic diuretics were as good or superior to newer drugs),[4] is not even on their radar screens. The result is that regulators allow physicians to become the unwitting accomplices of drug industry door-to-door salesmen who peddle not the most effective medicines, but those that are best for their firm's bottom line.

The tools for shifting the ground in this debate are starting to become available. Medical economists have begun comparing various medical interventions based not just on the amount of time that they add to a patient's life, but on the quality of that time. If broadly adopted by healthcare financers, this criterion will enable patients, as well as their physicians and insurers, to know that their healthcare decisions are based on criteria that give an appropriate weighting not only to "years to life" but also "life to years." In a world where medical technologies can keep a brain-dead Terry Schiavo alive for a decade, how long can we avoid making such judgments?

Over and over again in these pages, however, you will see that ubiquitous conflicts of interest stand in the way of applying these more rational approaches to the practice of medicine. The drug and medical device industries come in for a lot of criticism, all of it well deserved. Their relentless pursuit of profit from their proprietary products is threatening to undermine the scientific underpinnings of the practice of medicine, which has been more than a century in the making. Physicians and "key opinion leaders" who are padding their incomes by consulting or giving speeches on behalf of medical providers need to rethink where they are leading their profession.

The time has come for everyone involved in the delivery of healthcare – and that includes patients – to insist that objective evaluations of all the possible healthcare interventions inform the practice of medicine. This empirical evidence must be generated by medical scientists who are unencumbered by the blinders of financial conflicts of interest. Far more than the fiscal health of nations is at stake. Continued improvements in the health of advanced industrial societies will depend on making the changes suggested in this insightful book.

Merrill Goozner
Center for Science in the Public Interest
Washington DC
USA
December 2006

References

1 Cannon CP (2005) The IDEAL cholesterol: lower is better. *JAMA.* **294**: 2492–4.
2 de Lorgeril M, Salen P, Martin J, Monjaud I, Delaye J, Mamelle N (1999) Mediterranean diet, traditional diet, and the rate of cardiovascular complications after myocardial infarction: final report of the Lyon Heart Study. *Circulation.* **99**: 779–85.
3 Goozner M (2004) *The $800 Million Pill: the truth behind the cost of new drugs.* University of California Press, Berkeley, CA.
4 The ALLHAT Officers and Coordinators for the ALLHAT Collaborative Research Group (2002) Major outcomes in high-risk hypertensive patients randomized to angiotensin-converting enzyme inhibitor or calcium channel blocker vs diuretic: the antihypertensive and lipid-lowering treatment to prevent heart attack trial (ALLHAT). *JAMA.* **288**: 2981–97.

Author addresses

Cornelia J. Baines MD FACE
Professor Emerita
Department of Public Health Sciences
Room 401C
University of Toronto
155 College Street
Toronto
ON N5T 3M7
Canada
E-mail: cornelia.barnes@utoronto.ca

Patricia A. Baird OC OBC FRSC MD CM FRCPC FCCMG
Department of Medical Genetics
University of British Colombia
Wesbrook Building
6174 University Boulevard
Vancouver
BC V6T 1ZE
Canada
E-mail: pbaird@interchange.ubc.ca

Audrey Balay-Karperien MS
E-mail: akarpe@sbcglobal.net

Luc Bonneux PhD
Federal Health Care Knowledge Center
Brussels.
Belgium
E-mail: luc.bonneux1@telenet.be

Alan Cassels CD MPA
School of Health Information Sciences
University of Victoria
423 Stannard Avenue
Victoria
BC V8S 3M6
Canada
E-mail: alan@alancassels.com

Joy Fraser PhD RN
Centre for Nursing and Health Studies
Athabasca University
Athabasca
Alberta T9S 3A3
Canada
E-mail: joyf@athabascau.ca

Danny George MSc
Room 2-48
Graduate Centre
Hertford College
Folly Bridge
Oxford
OX1 4LA UK
E-mail: dgeorge2844@yahoo.com

Merrill Goozner MS
Integrity in Science
Center for Science in the Public Interest
1875 Connecticut Avenue
NW #300
Washington DC 20009
USA
E-mail: mgoozner@cspinet.org

Iahn Gonsenhauser MBA
Department of Neurology
Case Western Reserve University
University Memory and Aging Center
12200 Fairhill Road c355
Cleveland
OH 44120
USA
E-mail: ixg19@yahoo.com

Joel Lexchin MD
School of Health Policy and Management
York University
4700 Keele Street
Toronto
ON M3J 1P3
Canada
E-mail: jlexchin@yorku.ca

Donald W. Light PhD
Fellow, Netherlands Institute for Advanced Study
University of Medicine and Dentistry of New Jersey
10 Adams Drive
Princeton
NJ 08540
USA
E-mail: dlight@princeton.edu

Norman J. Temple PhD
Centre for Science
Athabasca University
Athabasca
Alberta T9S 3A3
Canada
E-mail: normant@athabasca.ca

Andrew Thompson PhD
Obere Weid 2
4125 Riehen
Switzerland
E-mail: Andrew.thompson@bluewin.ch

Peter J. Whitehouse MD PhD
Department of Neurology
Case Western Reserve University
University Hospitals of Cleveland
University Memory and Aging Center
12200 Fairhill Road c357
Cleveland
OH 44120
USA
E-mail: peter.whitehouse@case.edu

Introduction

The annual expenditure by the USA on the military is truly enormous and exceeds the combined military expenditure of the next nine countries. What is perhaps more remarkable is that this expenditure is exceeded by a factor of three and a half by spending on healthcare. The share of Gross Domestic Product (GDP) taken by healthcare in the USA is over 15%. Indeed, in most developed countries healthcare spending constitutes the largest single item of national expenditures. It is also the item that is most commonly out of control. Try as they may, developed countries have not been able to keep these costs from expanding. For decades annual increases in these expenditures in the world's wealthier countries have averaged close to 5% and there is no end in sight. In the USA, the country that leads the world in such expenditures, the share of the GDP cake taken by healthcare has trebled since 1960 (from just 5% to 15% and rising).

The extravagance on healthcare spending might be justified if we could see clear evidence that it was directly responsible for major gains in the health of populations, but there is scant evidence of this. Much of the modest increase in longevity in recent decades can be attributed to better living conditions and to people adopting a healthier lifestyle, such as less smoking. By contrast, increases in spending for remedial care, the expense-expanding factor, has played a much lesser role. We will give two examples to illustrate the point.

Starfield[1] documented the fact that in a ranking of 13 developed countries the USA came last for both infant mortality and low-birthweight percentages, and is in the bottom four for life expectancy at age 15. Overall, the USA ranked twelfth (one from the bottom) on average for the 16 available health indicators. Yet, in terms of health expenditure, the USA is head and shoulders above the rest. The explanation for this is the subject of some debate[2] but what is undeniable is that vast spending on healthcare does not translate into better health.

Another illustrative example is provided by changes in cancer patterns in recent decades. In the USA in 1930 stomach cancer killed ten times more people than did lung cancer, whereas today the numbers have been reversed.[3] One obvious explanation for this is the dramatic changes in diet and other aspects of lifestyle, especially smoking. By contrast, improvements in medicine have played a fairly minor role.

This is not to deny that modern medicine has improved the lot of many of us. Millions in the wealthier nations are in better health and suffer less because of new medical advances. In order to properly see the "big picture" we must recognize these successes of medicine. Examples of such therapeutic successes in recent decades include improved drug therapy for hypertension, cures for some forms of cancer common in children, and advances in treatment of traumatic injury. But, on balance, medicine has promised far more than it has delivered, and it seems impotent in so many areas. For example, in recent years there has been a pandemic of obesity sweeping the Western world. Medicine has spent decades fighting the "battle of the bulge," but with virtually no success.

It is safe to assume that if things carry on as they are the rapid upward trajectory of spending will continue for many years to come. The increasing frequency of obesity makes it inevitable that related diseases, such as type 2 diabetes, will become more prevalent in coming years. We can confidently predict that the aging of the many millions of baby boomers and the emergence of new drugs and technologies will ensure that the rise in the cost of medical care continues for years to come. New medical interventions often use high-tech expensive equipment and require highly trained personnel. One need only think of diagnosis using magnetic resonance imaging (MRI) or computerized axial tomography (CAT) scans. Intensive marketing, such as direct-to-consumer advertising of drugs, is also adding to rising medical costs.

Everyone involved in modern medicine is very conscious that spending is fast increasing. The reasons for this are manifold. And there are also many proposed strategies for regaining control. Each expert has his favorite axe to grind: more efficient management models; more government regulation and less open market competition (or vice versa); more preventive and less remedial care; converting to a one-payer system; to name a few. Most, perhaps all, the proposals have some merit to them, and a judicious combination of some of them could lead to reduction in growth of expenditures, perhaps even some temporary reductions. However, in this book we will be viewing the problem of healthcare spending from a radically different perspective.

So what has gone wrong? We are reminded of the words of Robert Frost: "We are making great progress, but we're headed in the wrong direction."

A key problem with modern medicine is that it has set itself off from all other concerns. It has convinced itself that what it offers is so important that other concerns will just have to take care of themselves. It is not its problem if many people lack basic food, shelter, sanitation, and education, and that our basic provider, the environment in which we live, is dying. Modern medicine does not seem concerned with the suffering that results from these lacks, albeit every bit as chronic and intense. Instead, it maintains its narrow focus on such pursuits as the need to develop more gene-targeted and mood-targeted drugs, and placing self-replicating neurons where they are needed, and then, somehow, everything will be much better, even though this pursuit drains the public coffers.

A few numbers will illustrate the extent of the imbalance. Here are the annual expenditures in Canada by the federal government for several important areas (costs are in Canadian dollars for 2004 or 2005):

- Preserving the natural environment and addressing climate change: $1000 million.[4]
- Canadian National Parks. These have some of the world's most spectacular scenery, such as Lake Louise, and are home to many endangered species, such as grizzly bears: $533 million.[5]
- CBC radio. This corporation provides a radio service free of advertising: $337 million.[6]
- Arts and culture: $172 million.[4]
- Sport: $140 million.[4]
- Foreign aid: $680 million.[4]

On top of this we can add the cost of public libraries of $967 million (based on Edmonton, extrapolated to the rest of Canada).[7]

This adds up to $3.8 billion. Without this spending on these seven essential areas Canada would be seriously devalued and quality of life would significantly deteriorate. By contrast, spending on prescription drugs, which is roughly one-fifth of total medical spending, was $18 billion in 2004.[8] This means that for every dollar spent on the above seven important areas, nearly five dollars goes on prescription drugs.

These numbers reveal that medicine sees itself as entitled to a huge slice of the national budgetary cake, and the government concedes by its actions that this is acceptable. Fortunately, there are notable exceptions in the medical world to this mind-set. Two organizations of physicians that stand out are Médicins sans Frontiers and Physicians for Social Responsibility. The former, especially, is sensitive to the importance of environmental factors such as pollution, and both are sensitive to the need for more emphasis on education, nutrition, and low-cost, basic preventive and remedial care. But the reality of the USA today is that millions do not have access to timely medical care, or to the more important life-extending and life-enhancing needs of proper nutrition, shelter, protection from toxic substances, and an education that would enable them to cope with modern life in all its complexities. We live in a "rob Peter to pay Paul" world and continuing very expensive pursuits into the understanding and cure of human diseases, fascinating and financially rewarding as these may be for some individuals and parts of our economy, is a death knell for others.

Another major factor that causes waste and extravagant spending within the healthcare system is conflict of interest. In recent years much evidence has accumulated that clearly reveals how commercial interests, in particular in the pharmaceutical industry, use their financial clout to influence all aspects of decision making.

One of the propositions argued in this book is that medicine should have no more resources than are justified, taking into account the many desperately under-funded demands on the national wealth. In summary, our goal is to replace the current "Rolls Royce medicine" with the development of a "VW medicine." To accomplish this, certain changes are highly desirable. Most of these have, at least in part, already been recommended by others. What is new is the packaging of them into a viable totality. Much of this work has already been broached in our previous book, *Ethics, Medical Research and Medicine*.[9] In this book we have further developed these proposals.

There is the necessity for confronting the question of cost head on, rather than considering it as an obstacle to be ignored wherever possible or to be overcome by political pressure. This confrontation must begin, where possible, at the research stage, since once a treatment is developed and approved for distribution, modern marketing practices make it highly likely that the profession and the public will demand that it be made available to all who might profit from it, regardless of cost. Estimates therefore need to be made as to how much a treatment is likely to cost, if it were to be fully developed. Such estimates could be made at several points in the research, but certainly before a lot of money is spent. If it becomes apparent that the research will result in a therapy that will likely exceed reasonable limits, given the society's total set of priorities, it will not receive any further public funding. In some cases, this will be clear before the research even starts. Currently, limits fluctuate according to who mounts the most successful campaign to get public funding for their research and treatments; the most powerful lobbies usually win out. Notice, we refer only to limits on public funding. This is because it is impractical to try to limit private individuals or groups from amassing and expending funds for the research and interventions they deem important. Some types of specific limits will be suggested, limits tailored to the society. Companion to this is the focus on seeking ways to improve the distribution of care that we already know is efficacious and affordable.

An essential change is the implementation, system-wide, of measures to combat the unholy alliance of personal profit and career-enhancement that infects all levels of modern medicine, from choice of research program to approval and promotion of new interventions.

Companion to this change is the implementation of a far more rigorous system for evaluating the worth of any new interventions, whether a new surgical procedure, a new screening test, or a new use for a drug. What happens now is that procedures may become established on the basis of hope and low-grade evidence for their efficacy, and then gain organizational support for campaigns to make them standard, recommended offerings. It can even be considered unethical to subject them to rigorous criteria since that would deny some patients the chance to benefit from them. But the only sure thing about their effect is that the medical conglomerate makes a profit from using them.

We will illustrate how the implementation of these changes could lead to tremendous savings in several high-cost areas of medical practice. These are screening for cancer, genetic research and therapy and use of statins. Directing our resources to preventive-care programs would do far more for our health.

We make no claim to having drawn a roadmap of how policies should be implemented. Rather, we are talking in general principles. Of course, the details will vary from country to country.

In sum, we offer a proposal for a revolution in medicine based on a paradigm that integrates medical care into the world as a whole rather than one that accords it a special status.

Andrew Thompson
University of Oregon (retired)
USA

Norman J. Temple
Athabasca University
Canada
December 2006

References

1 Starfield B (1998) *Primary Care: balancing health needs, services, and technology.* Oxford University Press, New York.
2 Starfield B (2000) Is US health really the best in the world? *JAMA.* **284**: 483–5.
3 Greenlee RT, Murray T, Bolden S, Wingo PA (2000) Cancer statistics, 2000. *Ca 2000.* **50**: 7–33.
4 Government of Canada (2005) Budget 2005. Available from www.fin.cg.ca/budtoce/2005/budliste.htm (accessed December 2, 2005).
5 Parks Canada (2005) Corporate Plan 2005. Available from www.parkscanada.ca (accessed September 29, 2005).
6 CBC (2005) CBC Annual Report, 2005. Available from www.edmonton.ca/CityGov/annualreports/budget/2003-2004 (accessed September 29, 2005).
7 City of Edmonton (2005) Edmonton Budget, 2005. Available from www.edmonton.ca/CityGov/corpservs/budget_2005 (accessed September 29, 2005).

8 Morgan S (2005) Canadian prescription drugs costs surpass 18 billion dollars. *Can Med Assoc J.* **172**: 1323–4.

9 Thompson A, Temple NJ (2001) *Ethics, Medical Research and Medicine: commercialization versus social justice and environmentalism.* Kluwer, Dordrecht.

Chapter 1

The cost of medical care: how much is too much?

Andrew Thompson and Norman J. Temple

The problem

The constant upward spiral in medical spending is well known and was briefly described in the Introduction. We will again illustrate the problem by giving some hard numbers:

- General Motors estimates that its healthcare expenses add $1400 to the cost of a new car.[1]
- It is projected that healthcare spending in the USA will exceed two trillion dollars in 2006.[2]
- The number of Americans without healthcare insurance has been steadily climbing and in 2003 reached 45 million.[3]
- According to US government figures the number of its citizens living in poverty has also been climbing and in 2004 reached 37 million, or one in every eight people. Even worse, almost 18% of children live in poverty.[4]

The enormous cost of healthcare in the USA is paid for in diverse ways, such as through taxes, insurance premiums, and higher prices for all goods and services. The inevitable result is that this spending drains money from other vital needs. And with the national purse under strain it is scarcely surprising if millions more people find themselves living in poverty and having only limited access to the medical system.

While the USA is clearly the leader in runaway healthcare expenditures, this problem is present across the Western world. In Canada, healthcare spending per capita by the government (in constant 1997 Canadian dollars) has almost doubled in the last 30 years: from $1257 in 1975–1976 to $2356 in 2005–2006 (forecast spending).[5]

Each year medical care eats up a slightly higher proportion of the budget. One reason for this is that there are no formal, ethically set limits of how much a government should spend. What limits that exist reflect the political climate at the time and are primarily the result of pressure from industrial, medical, and citizen lobbies. Medical research and treatment are routinely portrayed as crucial, life-saving activities, which elected officials dare not appear to be less than enthusiastic about. On the contrary, it is a way to gain public favor, and politicians loudly align themselves with campaigns for more research money to counter high-profile diseases, such as breast cancer and AIDS. In the face of such powerful forces it is difficult to carve out what is right, as opposed to what the majority and the powerful want.

One of the results of the present system is that a sizeable part of medical spending is directed to treatments and other medical procedures that were never properly tested and have not been proven of value, even if they have become widely accepted. As we shall see in later chapters, treatments of dubious value are all too common.

Calculating the value of medical interventions

Before we proceed farther in our discussion of reasonable cost limits for medical interventions, we first need to discuss how such costs can be best calculated. The challenge is to use a rational system so that diverse interventions can be compared in a meaningful way. An accepted way this can be done is based on a quality-adjusted life year, a QALY. The investigator calculates not only the number of extra years of life that a medical intervention delivers but also their quality. Quality of life is on a scale from 0 (death) to 1 (perfect physical health and being perfectly satisfied with life); in other words, from six feet under to *Baywatch*. It must be emphasized that with many medical interventions, such as rehabilitation after a heart attack or stroke, the extended years of lives are usually of diminished quality. This therefore increases the true cost of the intervention when expressed as dollars per QALY.

Evaluations of the real cost of medical interventions are often inaccurate because they are based, not on QALYs, but simply on life-years gained (LYG). LYGs give equal value to a year of life gained by someone who is restored to full health and another person who is alive but debilitated. It should be self-evident that it is more meaningful to measure medical outcomes as QALYs rather than as LYGs. One reason for the failure to use QALY is that there is no generally accepted measure of quality of life resulting from the intervention. This problem adds to the challenge of evaluating various medical interventions objectively, including several of those discussed in this book.

Here are some illustrative examples of using QALY. We start with Person A, who has a painful condition that is not life-threatening – arthritis, for example. While the treatment may add no years to Person A's life, it should increase the quality of those years. Accordingly, we can estimate the increased quality that should be gained and calculate the cost as dollars per QALY. If Person A is 50, and the treatment increases quality of life from 0.7 to 0.9, and assuming that his life expectancy is 80, the number of QALYs generated by treatment is 30 x 0.2 (i.e. [80–50] x [0.9–0.7]), or 6. (This is an illustrative example; in reality, Person A's physical health will decline as he ages.)

Let us now compare two people with cancer: Person B has an intervention that treats early-stage cancer while Person C has a treatment for advanced cancer. We must include in our estimations of dollars per QALY that the extra years of life of Person B are likely to be of much higher quality than those of Person C. Indeed, with Person C, and with many others who have suffered serious trauma or illness, the quality of life posttreatment may be very low, with much pain or disability. Clearly, this type of calculation is a very inexact science. In particular, putting a value on quality of life will vary considerably from person to person for reasons such as religious beliefs and self-perception of satisfaction with life.

The great advantage of measuring the real cost of medical interventions on the basis of dollars per QALY is that it allows a straightforward comparison of medical interventions that extend life and those that improve its quality. In effect, adding years to life and adding life to years are each given appropriate weight without irrationally throwing resources at one at the expense of the other.

When calculating QALY, as with so many other problems, the devil is in the detail. Analyses of the cost of medical interventions can be calculated in a variety of ways, some of which are questionable. For example, you can lower the cost of a procedure by subtracting from it an estimate of how much benefit was gained in work productivity of those treated. But, to be consistent, you should then also add to it the amount of time lost from work in order to have the procedure done, whether it is a screening for cancer, a laboratory test, or what have you. The result of these acts of creative accounting is often to reduce the apparent cost of medical procedures. Leaving out the cost of setting up and administrating a new procedure also has this effect.

Perhaps the most questionable estimates are those of the medical costs that have been avoided as a result of the intervention. For example, the estimated cost of screening for cancer can be lowered by deducting the cost of future cancer treatment that has now been avoided. The problem is that such savings are mostly, if not entirely, illusionary, given probable future medical costs. We can illustrate this by considering screening for breast cancer. Let us assume that for every 100 women who would die from breast cancer without screening, 20 will now avoid death from the disease. As a result the medical system will now be saved the high costs of treating these 20 women for terminal breast cancer. But these women will not disappear and never return to a hospital or clinic. Instead, most of them will survive into their seventies, during which time they will probably require treatment for any number of costly medical conditions, such as stroke or senility. So from a strictly economic point of view the estimated savings by avoiding treatment for cancer are likely to be false. The same is true for any intervention that prevents heart disease or any other fatal disease. Again, the effect of current practice is to artificially lower the estimated costs of the intervention. Ignoring these costs is rather like a company banking its employees' pension contributions but making no allowance for future pension payments.

Another source of error that reduces apparent costs is to assume that all those whose deaths from a particular disease have been prevented will now live full life spans. This is not realistic given that diseases do not attack randomly but tend to cluster together. They primarily target people who follow an unhealthy lifestyle or have other risk factors for disease. Such people – smokers, diabetics, and those raised in poverty, for example – are vulnerable to numerous deadly or debilitating diseases and conditions which may shorten the length and decrease the quality of their lives, irrespective of the intervention. It follows, therefore, that when a medical intervention prevents death from a particular disease, the beneficiaries will, on average, have a below average life span.

Unfortunately, cost-effectiveness models very often hide from the reader's eye the assumptions that have been made during the estimation. Our reading of many published reports leads us to strongly suspect that the factors given above are usually calculated inappropriately; the result of this is to seriously underestimate the cost per QALY. A related problem is that cost estimations are notorious for their wide ranges. Our aim here is to be as transparent as possible in whatever cost calculations we make.

What limits should be placed on the cost of medical treatment?

How much should a country's public coffers pay for the medical care of its citizens? This is one of the most difficult issues that face those who are the guardians of the fiscal health of every country. And, indeed, if one looks at the decision-making process, politicians and other public authorities rarely face up to it squarely. The amount spent on medical care becomes a political process subject to many ethical distortions. The task of setting an ethical limit means entering a moral quagmire, while imposing it means confronting powerful entrenched forces. Yet, to ignore this imposing task is to invite even more disastrous underfunding of every other worthy endeavor. Better to light a candle than curse the darkness.

The simple fact is that the laws of arithmetic dictate that a dollar spent in one place is a dollar unavailable elsewhere. For this reason we need to adopt firm cost limits for public funding of medical care. We have to determine what is truly worthy of being funded and what is not. Accordingly, firm limits need to be imposed and there must be an end to public funding for medical care that costs too much.

We begin our examination with a look at the existing, informal cost limits in the country that leads the world in many ways in such matters, the USA. During the 1970s Medicare decided to cover the cost of dialysis for chronic renal failure. The cost at that time worked out to $50 000 per QALY[6] and this became a benchmark. This limit has drifted upwards, but at a speed slower than inflation, so that nowadays a range of $50 000 to $100 000 per QALY is often cited as the cost limit. However, this figure is routinely ignored when spending decisions are taken. The actual limit followed by real doctors and real administrators is thought to be considerably higher, but there has been little serious discussion or investigation as what that limit really is.

Often a rule seems to be in operation that cost limits simply do not exist: no one will be denied a treatment that might benefit them, regardless of cost (provided, of course, they are eligible for coverage). The implications of this quasi-policy are well illustrated by the case of the left ventricular assist device. Medicare opted to pay for its use despite its estimated cost-effectiveness being between $500 000 and $1.4 million per QALY.[7] This situation is the inevitable result when a system refuses to contemplate cost limts.

The UK appears to have limits (translated to 2005 US dollars) of around $50 000 per QALY.[6] It is therefore apparent that the USA and the UK have a wide divergence in their spending limits.

In the USA the actual cost limits for medical interventions are determined by the interaction of many agencies, from federal governments down to local governments. For those who have private insurance, the limits are set by the healthcare plans of third-party insurers, and each insurer decides what procedures it will cover. These companies, in competition with each other, strive to cover what the public is most apt to want to see in a plan, almost regardless of its cost, and try to economize by cutting back elsewhere.

Governments at various levels in the USA are generally in a strong position to influence spending limits as they pay over half of medical costs.[8] First, they can determine how much they will pay for those groups whose medical costs are paid directly by government, such as their own employees and the retired. Second, they can influence what private firms and practitioners can charge particular groups of people. We can see, therefore, that governments have the means for enacting reasonable and ethical limits for medical spending.

This influence begins quite early in the process. The likely cost of a proposed treatment can often be estimated while the treatment is still at the research stage. A decision can then be taken that if that cost is higher than the allowed limit, then no public funding will be provided for either further development or for any treatment that may result from it. And another important stage occurs when an application is made for approval of the procedure or product. It is vitally important to ensure that it passes a rigorous examination of its efficacy, and this should include an analysis of cost-effectiveness. What is necessary, however, is the political will to do so.

This brings us back to the question: What should be the ethical limit for public expenditures on medical treatment? To help determine this we have to take into account that health is just one of many values that should be promoted in a society. Many might argue that health is the most important because without it life would not be worth living. But health is clearly not the only determinant of what makes life worth living. Indeed, many people with serious impairments can accomplish much and live what they consider a satisfactory life, or at least one they would want to continue. Other factors also widely considered to be of much value include satisfaction with accomplishments, good relations with family and others, broadening of knowledge and understanding, seeing the unfolding of nature, and the observance of religious belief. Indeed, there are many ways to enhance the quality of life, such as money spent on assisting the underpriviledged and reducing pollution. How we prioritize these aspects of living is obviously a matter of value judgment.

Given all these objectives, the danger is that in the battle for the available resources, the ones that predominate will be those from which most profit can be made. And, for some time, the big winner has been the medical industry – the vast conglomerate of researchers, developers of products and procedures and their stock owners, practitioners, and private healthcare insurers. This is clearly shown by the amount of money and other resources consumed by the industry. The result is that other concerns, based on other values, receive a smaller slice of the pie.

Let us take a different, even broader, approach to answering the above question. Let us say that the most important value is to promote the possibility that everyone, as far as is reasonably possible, has the maximum chance to achieve a full, satisfying life, however they would define it. John Stuart Mill expressed this sentiment thus: "The greatest good for the greatest number." "Governments of the people and for the people," in so far as such exist, can be said to strive to achieve this utilitarian goal for their citizens.

Let us now look at different ways to approach the question of cost limits for medical interventions. This will take the form of cost cut-off points in terms of dollars per QALY. Clearly, this should be dramatically less than what the current system in the USA allows. But at this point in the story a major challenge presents itself: any cost limit is, in reality, little more than a value judgment. We strongly suspect that had we commissioned a dozen top experts on medical ethics and health economics, we would have ended up with a dozen different numbers spread right across the map. In the discussion below, the two authors of this chapter present their estimations of appropriate cost limits.

Approach 1 (AT)

As a beginning point I propose that the upper limit for a medical intervention should not exceed the average annual expenditures of members of a society. This indicates how much it costs to live an average life in that society. In the USA, in 2001–2002, the average total of expenditures of a single person was $23 850.[9] A corresponding amount in 2005 dollars would be about $25 500. I propose, therefore, that the cost limit be $25 500 per QALY. Should this prove too high to allow coverage of all societal members, it should be lowered if the missing funding is not obtained by trimming the excessive costs of current products and procedures.

Approach 2 (NT)

I will base my estimation on what can reasonably be described as "affordable" for real, average people. I shall start with a rather average two-person family. They live in Edmonton, a city located in Alberta, Canada. This city has a standard of living comparable to the North American average. Their combined income is $60 000 (Canadian dollars) and this will give them a monthly take-home pay of about $3800. For purposes of simplicity I will assume that the couple are in perfect health. I shall now imagine two hypothetical disease situations. One day Mrs Average suddenly develops a strange metabolic disorder. Without treatment, she will be dead in a month. Fortunately, there is a treatment, Drug X, which will restore her to full health, but only if she takes it every day for the rest of her life. Now the question is: What is the maximum this family should reasonably pay for supplies of Drug X? No doubt, both Mrs Average and her loving husband would consider no amount too high. After all, we are talking life and death. And that is the great difficulty in setting cost limits: it is all too easy to be overcome by emotion. So we will step backward and try to answer the question using some cold hard numbers. I will start by assuming that Drug X is only available if paid for by Mr and Mrs Average out of their own money. After all, if the concept of "affordability" means anything, it should mean that average people can afford it. So the question now becomes: What is the maximum that Mr and Mrs Average can afford for supplies of Drug X? Naturally, they are prepared to make every sacrifice to afford the drug. So they decide that one of them will get a second job and they will reduce their living standards down to the poverty level. That means that their net income has increased to about $4600 while their expenses have fallen to about $1600 (fortunately for them, housing in Edmonton is cheaper than in many other cities). That allows them to pay up to $3000 per month for the drug, or $36 000 per year. For large numbers of people, this amount would actually be appreciably less; if the couple had a low income, if they had children, or they lived in a city where housing was more expensive, then the maximum that could be afforded for the drug would shrink to as little as zero. Therefore, based on this estimation of how much real people can afford, the maximum cost of one QALY should be no more than CAN$36 000 or US$31 000.

But what if the disease were debilitating rather than fatal? To answer this question I shall imagine that Mr Average is sideswiped by migraine. His condition is so painful that his quality of life is reduced by 20%, from 1 to 0.8. Here again a treatment is available: Drug Y. How much is our couple prepared to pay for the drug? There is no obvious answer to this question but somewhere around $500 per month seems a fair guess. This translates to a value for one QALY of around

CAN\$30 000 (i.e. \$500 x 12 [months] x 5 [quality of life rises by 0.2]), or about US\$26 000. Some people in the same situation would, no doubt, be prepared to spend more, perhaps twice as much.

I have now made two estimates, based on my average Edmonton couple, of an appropriate cost limit for medical expenditures, namely \$31 000 and \$26 000 per QALY. I could repeat this exercise with different scenarios in the USA, but I would expect the result to look rather similar. I again stress that these estimates are subject to many variables and therefore others might easily arrive at bottom lines that are double or half these figures.

We have now made three estimates of an appropriate cost limit for medical expenditures in the USA, namely \$25 500, \$31 000 and \$26 000 por QALY. Clearly, although the approaches were very different, the bottom lines were reasonably close. Let us now take a rough average: a cost limit of \$27 000 per QALY. If implemented, our proposed limit would sharply reduce healthcare spending since many medical interventions presently in use cost far in excess of this amount.

From a practical perspective, it should be acknowledged that it will be very difficult to institute any limit below \$50 000 per QALY in the USA, at least in the foreseeable future. Indeed, there are some expensive practices that are so well-entrenched that the public may be extremely reluctant to give them up. As of now, a large portion of the public can be expected to join the medical industry in opposing any restriction, adding to the industry's already overwhelming clout due to its full coffers and political influence. However, the voices of those who have developed doubts about the present medical paradigm and its societal impact are starting to be heard. If nothing else, economic considerations may well prompt a rethinking of the sacred status of remedial medicine in the current priority system.

The present system relies on physicians to control costs, but physicians are pressured in many ways to prescribe "the best possible care" to all, which often means the most expensive. Physicians must therefore not be given the option to choose overly expensive interventions. As Richard Lamm[10] noted, "You cannot build an ethical code for a publicly funded system around the assumption that 'cost is never a consideration' and that the focus of moral concern must be solely on the individual."

Based on this assessment we can now propose a twin set of cost limits. A medium-term goal is \$50 000 per QALY, whereas the lower limit, \$27 000, should be seen as both an ideal limit and a longer-term goal. We must again emphasize that both these figures are very rough estimates and open to debate.

These limits should be imposed on public funding of medical practice. The limits should also apply to research programs and product development: these should not be funded with taxpayers' money if the new medical procedure being developed is expected to cost in excess of these limits. However, as this discussion is limited to the public purse, no limit can or should be imposed on individuals or organizations who wish to purchase more expensive interventions.

Conclusion

Clearly, there is a yawning gap between expenditures deemed reasonable for normal living or affordable by average people and those deemed acceptable for medical procedures. It is as if the medical world is divorced from society and is living on another, far more opulent planet. The public, in effect, spends lavishly on medical care at the expense of its overall welfare.

The result of this is that large sections of the population become limited in their ability to afford things such as higher education, culture, and the many other activities that are needed in order to lead a satisfying life, while a minority reap handsome benefits as a result of this priority system. Governments are often accused of wasting large amounts of taxpayers' money in various ways. But it must be stressed that because medical care is so demanding of resources, it has far more impact than any other form of governmental excessive spending. This only makes the situation worse for all other societal needs. The most direct way to begin to correct this spending crisis is to set and enforce upper limits for those components of medical care that are to be subsidized from public coffers. Our proposed cost limits are a medium-term goal of $50 000 per QALY, while a lower limit, $27 000, should be seen as both an ideal limit and a longer-term goal.

References

1   Institute for America's Future (2004) Wal-Mart, General Motors may use Bush Plan to cut health costs. Citing *Bloomberg News*, September 27, 2004. Available from www.ourfuture.org (accessed November 6, 2005).
2   Centers for Medicare & Medicaid Services (2004) *National Health Expenditures and Selected Economic Indicators, Levels and Average Annual Percent Change: selected calendar years 1990–2013, January*. Available from www.cms.hhs.gov/statistics/nhe/projections-2003/t1.asp (accessed November 6, 2005).
3   DeNavas-Walt C, Proctor B, Mills RJ (2004) *Income, Poverty, and Health Insurance Coverage in the United States: 2003*. US Census Bureau, Washington, DC.
4   Wolf R (2005) *USA Today*, 30 August. Available from www.usatoday.com/news/washington/2005–08–30-census-poverty_x.htm (accessed November 12, 2005).
5   Canadian Institute for Health Information (2005) *Preliminary Provincial and Terrirorial Government Health Expenditure Estimates: 1974–1975 to 2004–2005*. Canadian Institute for Health Information, Ottowa.
6   Neumann PJ (2005) *Using Cost-effectiveness Analysis to Improve Health Care*. Oxford University Press, Oxford.
7   Gillick MR (2004) Medicare coverage for technological innovations – time for new criteria? *N Engl J Med* **350**: 2199–203.
8   Lamm RD (2004) The elephant in the living room of the house of health care. *American Journal of Bioethics* **4**: 101–2.
9   Bureau of Labor Statistics (2004) Table 3600. Consumer units of one person by age of reference person: average annual expenditures and characteristics, Consumer Expenditure Survey, 2001–2002. Available from www.bls.gov/ro5 (accessed August 24, 2004).
10 Lamm RD (1999) Redrawing the ethics map. *Hastings Cent Rep* **29**: 28–9.

Chapter 2

The nuts and bolts of medical research

Norman J. Temple and Andrew Thompson

Introduction

In this chapter we review how medical research is done. Many readers, no doubt, will already be familiar with this important subject. But others may find it helpful so that they can better judge the value of reports published in the medical literature or the popular media about medical findings. What is the noise-to-signal ratio? Does the new "discovery" give us good reason to be hopeful?

Types of research study

Epidemiological studies

Over the last several decades an enormous amount of valuable information has been gained by a form of research called epidemiology. Here the researcher looks for relationships between factors that people are exposed to (diet, lifestyle, environment), on on the one hand, and, on the other, health status and disease. This research strategy has led to a great many important findings; for example, people who drink alcohol in moderation or eat fish have less risk of heart disease; people exposed to passive smoking are at increased risk of lung cancer; and those who take little exercise are more likely to develop type 2 diabetes.

The first rule to understand about epidemiology is that it reveals "association not causation." So when we discover, for example, that the French drink plenty of red wine and have a relatively low level of heart disease, this means that red wine and heart disease are *associated* (in this case inversely associated). We must avoid the common mistake of jumping to the conclusion that the association is one of cause and effect, in this case that drinking red wine actually *prevents* heart disease.

Epidemiological studies are especially valuable in telling us how to prevent disease. Such studies generally have far less to say in the realm of therapy. However, with some conditions, heart disease for example, what applies to disease causation also applies to disease therapy. Thus, just as a diet overly rich in saturated fat causes heart disease, so a reduction in this food component is valuable in the treatment of that disease. We see similar examples in several other conditions, such as obesity, hypertension, and diabetes: findings from epidemiological studies have revealed a great deal about the causes of these conditions and this information also points to effective therapies.

This brings us to research on various types of treatment. Ideas for new treatments may come from diverse lines of investigation such as epidemiology, studies of disease mechanisms, from fishing expeditions looking for new chemicals with potentially useful actions in the body, or may be borrowed from herbal treatments. But regardless of where the idea came from, it is worth little until it has been proved to be effective. Here we look at the value of different types of studies into the effectiveness of treatments.

Studies on other animals

A large part of the research enterprise is conducted on other animals. When looking at results from such studies, it is best to keep in mind that even with our closest relatives, the primates, the differences between them and humans have been millions of years in the making. The favorite laboratory human substitutes, mice and rats, are considerably more distant, although claimed to be over 95% similar. This means that what is found to be curative for one of our animal relatives is often found not to be curative for us, or, if it is, the side effects may be more harmful than the cure is helpful. The reverse is true also: what is found to be ineffective or toxic in nonhumans may benefit humans. In fact, the only way to know with any confidence what is curative with a particular species is to experiment on that species. We have had more than a half a century of alleged cancer cures in mice and other substitute species that were going to revolutionize therapy, with essentially none living up to their headlined potential. Such studies spark interest but are not something that should inspire too much optimism.

Preliminary studies on humans

In terms of reliability the next step up from mice and rats is preliminary – or pilot – studies on small numbers of human volunteers. Such studies can indicate how much benefit, if any, is realized from a new treatment and therefore whether a larger study is justified. They also help determine the best design for a larger study, such as what dosage to give of the experimental substance and what problems a new treatment may pose. Preliminary studies also help to determine how many subjects are needed; for example, if a new treatment has only small advantages over an existing treatment, then a large number of subjects will be needed to clearly demonstrate this.

Because of their small size, preliminary studies are of limited value. However, those studies with promising findings are the ones most likely to get coverage, both in the medical literature as well as in the popular press, and this helps build a case for more funding and approval for further research.

Clinical trials

The gold standard for medical research is the randomized, controlled clinical trial (RCT). The RCT can be used in either prevention or therapy. It starts with the recruitment of subjects. Typically, these are healthy people at increased risk of a particular disease, in which case the researchers are testing whether an intervention will prevent that disease. Or the subjects may be patients who already have the disease of interest and the researchers are testing the efficacy of a new therapy.

RCTs have the following key features:

- Subjects (or patients) are divided into two or more groups randomly. The researchers ensure that groups are similar for obviously important variables, such as gender, by randomizing within these categories.
- The new treatment will be compared with either a placebo (dummy pills) or an existing treatment.
- When possible, neither the subjects nor the investigators know which subject is receiving which treatment (i.e. the study is double-blind).

There are important reasons why the selection of which subject receives what treatment is done randomly, not by choice of the subjects. Randomization of subjects has the great advantage that many variables that may be important, such as stress and social class, are likely to have a similar distribution in each group. Thus, at the end of the study, any differences in health between the two groups should be clearly attributed to the treatment rather than to some unknown factor X.

An RCT will include at least two groups, namely a treatment group and a control group (though other names may be used). The treatment group receives the new treatment being investigated while the control group receives either a placebo (and for that reason may be referred to as the placebo group) or an already-existing treatment. A placebo will appear identical to the treatment but has no active ingredient.

Double blinding is especially important. Think what would happen without it. First, the subjects are likely to react more positively if they know they are having an active treatment rather than an inactive one. Second, it is all too easy for the researchers to convey a more positive attitude to subjects in the group receiving the new experimental treatment (which the researchers may personally believe is a wonderful medical advance). And, third, the investigators may allow their biases to influence how they record the results of the study. With conditions such as arthritis and migraine it is all too easy to for the investigator to hear what he wants to hear when recording a patient's description of his level of pain and discomfort. Great care must therefore be taken to ensure in blinded studies that the code that identifies which treatment each patient is receiving is not revealed to team members during the study.

Sometimes the comparison is between obviously different procedures, for example invasive experimental surgery and a noninvasive procedure. In such cases it will be obvious to both the therapists and the subjects as to which group each subject is in, so there is no double blinding and the biases mentioned above are apt to appear.

Predictably, not everyone who enters an RCT is still actively involved at the end. The problem here is that those who choose to drop out may be quite different from those who stay the course and this can cause yet another source of bias. The extent of this problem has been much discussed in the medical press in recent years. As a result, a variety of guidelines have been developed. One is the commitment to analyze all of the results of all the participants in the study, regardless of whether they drop out or are dropped at some later time for one reason or another. This removes the temptation to eliminate participants who are in the intervention group but who are not benefiting. This procedure is referred to as "analysis by intention to treat."

That is the basis of the RCT. The problem is that many studies have failed to follow all these guidelines. In particular, we have good reasons for serious concern if double blinding is not done. But that does not mean that an RCT with double blinding will yield clear, unambiguous results. As we shall see, there are still many sources of bias.

Placebo or existing treatment: questions of ethics

A major concern with many RCTs which are investigating new therapies is whether the control group should receive a placebo or an existing treatment of proven efficacy for the condition or disease. The Food and Drug Administration (FDA) of the USA customarily accepts trial designs that test against a placebo. In fact, the FDA considers this trial design to be the "gold standard."[1] But this policy has a serious flaw. A new drug is considerably more likely to be found effective when compared to a placebo rather than to an existing drug. The reason for this is rather obvious: if the new drug has only a weak effect, comparison against a placebo will probably show a benefit whereas comparing it with an existing drug, which may actually be more potent, will probably show little or no advantage for the new drug. Use a placebo for the control group is, in effect, placing the goalposts where a "goal" can most easily be scored. This is both bad science and unethical. It is bad science as it may show merely that the new drug works but without answering the much more important question: Does it have an advantage over the existing drug? It is unethical as it means that the patients in the placebo group are not being given an effective treatment.

The pharmaceutical industry prefers a study design in which the control group receives a placebo rather than an existing treatment as this eases the path to approval of the new drug. In Canada, this study design is not allowed, except for very mild conditions, unless there is no established and effective treatment. So, for example, a trial carried out in Canada of a new medication for hypertension cannot include a placebo group as effective drugs are available for that condition. But as it is the USA that has the largest market for drugs in the world, its policies, and not Canada's, dominate how most drug research is done.

The opinion we prefer, and on which Canada's policy is based, is found in the following statement on human rights, as updated in 2002:

> *The benefits, risks, burdens and effectiveness of a new method should be tested against those of the best current prophylactic, diagnostic and therapeutic methods. This does not exclude the use of placebo, or no treatment, in studies where no proven prophylactic, diagnostic or therapeutic method exists. (From the World Medical Association Declaration of Helsinki, 2004)*[2]

Another problem with RCTs lies in recruiting volunteers. Many people are understandably reluctant to risk being assigned to the group given a placebo and still have to go to all the trouble of being periodically prodded, blood-sampled, urine-tested, or what have you. Other people may be fearful about being submitted to some experimental intervention without any guarantee that it will not lead to untoward side effects. Of course, RCTs are governed by strict ethical rules which stipulate that risks must be minimized and, as far as possible, communicated to the participants (i.e. they must give "informed consent"). But new treatments, by their very nature, involve much uncertainty. One would think that participants in RCTs should be paid for their efforts. But paying people invites a host of other problems which lack of space prevents us from going into, so in most cases the only reward that participants receive is the assurance that they are contributing to the advancement of medical science. For all these reasons recruiting enough participants is often quite difficult. Moreover, those who are recruited may very well not be typical of the target population for the new treatment. So here, too, the voluntary aspect of the research undermines the trustworthiness of the results.

Sources of error in clinical trials

Bias by researchers

Not only is the motivation of the participants important but so also is the motivation of the members of the research team. We therefore need to examine their true motives. Is their dominant aim to advance the cause of medical science, even if this means demonstrating that the new therapy is useless and that years of research and development were a waste of time and money? Or is there, perhaps, a strong element of wanting to make an important finding, one that will have benefits in realms such as career advancement and prestige in the scientific community, and perhaps even some financial reward? Such motives are all too human. They can affect all aspects of the study, beginning with the choice of the target of research, the design of the study, how it is conducted, and how it is written up. Most, if not all, key team members are going to want the experimental intervention to succeed, and they will certainly not want to see a worsening of the health of study subjects. Thus, given the chance, some of them may consciously or unconsciously tilt the results towards the favorable side. There are many ways of doing this, depending on the role of the people involved.

Commerce and medical research

One strong incentive that comes into play is that created by money and career interests. In some areas of research, such as drug development and genomic medicine, much of the funding now comes from private enterprise. Such research is first and foremost a commercial activity with the goal of discovering things that can be sold, whether in the form of information, procedures, or products. Typically, the product will be something that can be protected by a patent. This has led to legal battles to extend the scope of what can be patented to newly discovered genes and the knowledge of their functions. Sometimes, the company often does not even have to discover anything of real value, but just look as if it might, and considerable money can be made off the rise in its stock value.

Such commercial enterprises have moved into and, indeed, have now become a major driving force in much medical research. Their money has become an important source of revenue for university departments in biomedical areas. The acceptance of money and equipment and even specialized training from private companies can easily lead down a slippery slope where, eventually, the profit motive triumphs over truly beneficial research. Some universities establish their own private companies which actively pursue projects intended to produce royalties and patents. The motive for this is likely to be a desire to make a profit but without submitting to external control. But this in no way allows us to assume that the interests of the general public are being served. A further crumbling of the traditional role of university research is brought about by making academic advancement and tenure dependent, to a greater or lesser extent, on carrying out research that leads to financial reward for the department and the university.

Some of these sources of conflict of interests will be detailed in later chapters. The key point here is to appreciate some of the varied reasons for being cautious before accepting new medical findings at face value.

Sources of error in published reports

After an RCT has been carried out, it must then be written up as a paper and published. More distortions in research routinely occur at this stage.

How to make small differences look much larger

Most types of study on humans express their findings in a form called relative risk statistics. Here are some typical examples.

- Smoking increases the risk of lung cancer 20-fold.
- People with a relatively high consumption of cereal fiber have a 30% reduced risk of developing type 2 diabetes.
- Statins (a class of drugs that lower the blood cholesterol level) reduce the risk of dying from coronary heart disease (CHD) by one-third.

Now, in each case, expressing the results in this form has strong advantages. First, it is clear what the statements mean. Second, and very importantly, showing relative risk accords with what we typically find in research studies of this type, namely that relative risk is typically quite stable in very different situations,[3] it tends to change to only a small degree in different age groups, between men and women, and in those at high or low risk of the disease in question. So, for example, everything we know about statins suggests that everyone can reduce their risk of dying from CHD by about one-third if they take a statin every day.

So, as a means to report the findings of research studies, relative risk is the standard method. But, and this is a very serious "but," it does have a major limitation: it does not tell us how much actual benefit will be achieved by acting on the information. Indeed, relative risk can actually be quite misleading. We can illustrate this by considering the case of a man who is about to make two trips by car. First, he plans to drive to the store, a distance of one kilometer. And then he plans to drive 500 km. If he wears a seat belt while driving, this will reduce his risk of injury by approximately 70%, a fact that holds true in pretty much all circumstances. So on each trip, his relative risk of injury is reduced by 70% by wearing a seat belt. But, obviously, it is hundreds of times more likely that his seat belt will actually save him from injury on the long trip than on the short trip. This difference is so extreme that this man, after weighing the probabilities, may well decide not to bother to use his seat belt on the short trip but will be sure to use it on the long trip.

Now let us apply this principle to a medical situation. Suppose you read a report in a medical journal of a large RCT on patients with high cholesterol levels. The authors report that giving a statin reduces the risk of dying from CHD by one-third.

This sounds very impressive. The report may convince you that everyone whose cholesterol level is elevated should take the drug. But if you did so, you would be making the mistake of jumping to conclusions based on only half the story.

Let us now look at how the numbers are calculated. Suppose there were 1000 people in the group that took the statin and 1000 people in the control group that took the placebo. Sixty people died from CHD in the placebo control group and 40 in the statin group during the duration of the study (typically five years). Thus, the proportion who died from CHD was 60/1000, or 6%, of the placebo group and 40/1000, or 4%, of the statin group. As 4% is one-third less than 6%, one can therefore say that the drug reduced the risk of dying from CHD by one-third. This is "relative risk."

But, looking at the same numbers another way we see that, in reality, there was a reduction of only 2% in deaths from CHD (6% minus 4%). This far smaller reduction is called an "absolute risk reduction" and it gives a more meaningful picture of what actually happened with this particular group of patients. It shows that only 2% of the subjects who took statins actually avoided death from CHD as a result. Another way to provide a clear description of the results is to calculate the "number needed to treat" (NNT) in order for one person to benefit. It is 100 divided by the absolute risk reduction. In this example, it is 100 divided by 2, or 50. In other words, 50 people with high cholesterol have to take the statin for five years for one of them to benefit in terms of not dying from CHD.

The absolute risk reduction of 2% (or NNT of 50) tells us about patients of the type used in this study. This information is of practical value for doctors having to make clinical decisions. If the study had been carried out on subjects at only half the risk of death from CHD, the results would still have shown a relative risk reduction of about one-third (i.e. from 3% in the placebo group to 2% in the statin group). But, now, the absolute risk reduction is only half as strong (i.e. 1% [3% minus 2%] with a NNT of 100).

We see, therefore, that relative risk allows us to make statements of a general nature about statins; statements that apply to a wide range of people with equally wide differences in their actual risk of CHD. The reduction in absolute risk that we expect to see when patients are treated with statins depends on their level of risk: the higher their level of risk, the greater will be their reduction in absolute risk.

The way that numbers are presented has great importance when it comes to pharmaceutical companies providing meaningful information to doctors who must then explain this to their patients regarding treatment choices. Information given in terms of absolute risk reduction indicates the probability that the drug will actually prevent death from CHD for a particular type of patient. We will return to this question in a later chapter when we look at statins in more detail, but suffice to say that by basing treatment decisions on absolute risk, doctors can make treatment decisions in a more rational way; it helps them to avoid wasting expensive drugs on patients who are unlikely to benefit. Giving statins to patients at low risk of CHD is analogous to our car driver wearing a seat belt for a one kilometer drive (except that the former costs millions and the latter costs nothing). The same general points apply to a wide range of medical decision making.

It should now be clear that presenting the findings from a clinical study as relative risk can easily be misleading. Indeed, it is often a ploy so that the statistics deliver the desired message. When an advertisement for a drug claims that it will lower the risk of disease X by 30%, but without clearly explaining what the numbers really mean, this is a gross exaggeration of the benefit of the intervention.

It should come as little surprise that when it comes to giving warnings concerning the risk of adverse events, drug companies invariably choose the non-exaggerative way of describing the chances of something happening. For instance, people will be cautioned that there is, say, a one chance in a thousand risk of liver damage as a result of using statins. This is much more reassuring than being informed that the risk of this condition will increase by a factor of 100.

Problems in estimating risk of death

Many studies are done with the intention of demonstrating that the intervention prevents deaths from a particular disease. Ironically, the most important piece of information to the individual patient and the public is usually missing or buried in a difficult-to-decipher table in the report. It is the total number of people who died in each group, not just those who died of a particular disease, such as CHD or cancer, but those who died from any and all causes. The statistic indicating the total number of deaths is referred to as "all-cause mortality" or "overall mortality." This figure should tell us whether the treatment actually extends life. If the treatment extends lives among those with the target disease while also posing an acceptably low risk of side effects, then this should be indicated by the numbers for all-cause mortality. But if the treatment has side effects which act to shorten life, perhaps in ways that are multiple and diverse and thus not obvious, this may well be reflected in a failure of the treatment to reduce all-cause mortality.

There is a simple way of determining the actual likelihood of life extension. One keeps track of how many people in each group died during the time that they were studied; what they died of is irrelevant for the statistic. This estimation can be done accurately whereas determining an exact cause of death is more prone to error and more subject to bias.

All-cause mortality is the true test of any treatment that purports to be life-extending and is the only way to determine if the treatment really makes a difference. Who cares if deaths from heart attacks are prevented but the subjects die just as soon from something else? But people often make the mistake of assuming that if they are prevented from dying or are cured of one disease, they will live 10 or more years longer. However, having or being susceptible to a deadly disease could well be a sign that there is something wrong with the body's functioning which makes it vulnerable to other diseases and conditions. This becomes rather obvious with many elderly people who not only have heart disease but whose system is now under threat from decades of living an unhealthy lifestyle, such as smoking, and which might cause or contribute to their death. Therefore, reducing the likelihood of death from one cause does not mean that some other cause cannot and will not take its place. So a treatment might be successful in preventing risk of death from one disease but may bring about a disappointingly small decrease in the overall risk of death.

We must at this point recognize a distinction between what is ideal and what is feasible when it comes to measuring the impact of a medical intervention on risk of death. Let us start with a situation where all-cause mortality should certainly be a key outcome. In patients who have clinical CHD, death from this disease accounts for over half of all deaths. In the case of a treatment such as statins, in those patients where the claim is made that they will prevent CHD deaths, the study should be designed with enough patients so as to demonstrate both that deaths from CHD are reduced and also that all-cause mortality is reduced.

But things get considerably more challenging when we deal with diseases which account for only a small fraction of deaths, such as interventions designed to reduce risk of death from specific types of cancer. In later chapters we will be looking at whether screening for cancer is truly as beneficial as its proponents claim. Here, we shall briefly examine some of the problems involved in investigating this. Let us imagine that we have carried out a typical RCT of screening, namely the use of mammography for the prevention of death from breast cancer. In this RCT 30 000 women, aged 50–55, were randomized into two groups, each of 15 000: one group was given mammography and a control group received no intervention. After 15 years the findings reveal that there were 80 deaths from breast cancer in the group given mammography and 100 in the control group. So on the surface this looks like mammography has saved 20 women from death from breast cancer. But, alas, we must be hesitant before jumping to that conclusion; there are several sources of what may be significant error. Each group of women had a total of about 2000 deaths of which about 400 were due to cancer. With these numbers it would be quite easy to erroneously conclude that mammography had indeed prevented 20 deaths from breast cancer. This could be done by classifying 20 breast cancer deaths among women given mammography and call them deaths from another type of cancer, or by doing the reverse in the control group. Another source of error comes from possible harm done by the mammography itself. Suppose the X-rays caused 20 deaths from either heart disease or nonbreast cancer. This will almost certainly go unnoticed but would be enough to cancel out all the benefit from the breast cancer deaths prevented. So, even with the best of intentions, a narrow focus on deaths from breast cancer could easily generate a spurious conclusion. This problem is further discussed by Luc Bonneux in Chapter 11.

These sources of possible error should be considered when we are asked to accept that an RCT has shown a reduction in deaths from a particular cause. Is the reduction in deaths real or were the deaths prevented in one place cancelled out by extra deaths elsewhere? What it means is that we must be hesitant before accepting reports at face value. And in the case of screening for cancer this raises the possibility that the benefits may have been exaggerated.

How should researchers better design their RCTs so as to generate conclusions that inspire complete confidence? Unfortunately, there is no simple solution to this problem. Let us briefly review the choices. The obvious route is to compare all-cause mortality. In our study on breast cancer we could compare the total number of deaths in the two groups of women. Alas, this is a nonstarter: for reasons of statistics it is impossible to demonstrate that mammography has truly prevented 20 deaths from breast cancer among a total of 2000 deaths. In order to demonstrate that such a minute decrease is not due to chance it would require an impossibly large number of subjects in the study. One possible option is to determine which women are most at risk for the particular disease and study only them. If the intervention does not result in reduced all-cause deaths with even this population, then it is rather unlikely to do so with the general population.

In any case it is important that investigators in RCTs redouble their efforts to minimize the sources of error discussed above and design studies so the results stand up to close scrutiny. That means, first, that every effort must be made to accurately determine the cause of all deaths and, second, that possible adverse effects of interventions must be carefully investigated.

Reviews of clinical trials

So far we have looked at RCTs as single studies. However, when important treatments and medical interventions are being investigated, then several RCTs will most probably be performed. Differences will be seen between the results of each RCT. These can arise for any number of reasons; for example, random error or differences in the design of the studies, such as the type of subjects being studied. At this stage the results of the various RCTs are looked at collectively. The more studies combined together, and the greater the total number of subjects, the better the chances of forming an accurate picture of the real effect of the intervention.

Sometimes this can take the form of a simple review: the reviewer looks at each study separately and presents an expert opinion as to what it all means. Or this could be done in a rather more sophisticated manner: a systematic review. A trend in recent years is for researchers to obtain all the data from similar studies and merge them together, thereby creating what is, in effect, a jumbo-sized study. This is known as a "meta-analysis."

From clinical trials to medical practice

The whole object of the exercise thus far has been to determine if the new medical intervention is actually worth using. It is therefore of paramount importance to assess the evidence in its entirety. But, as should be apparent by now, there are many obstacles to coming to an accurate conclusion. And there are a few more challenges that we have not yet mentioned.

It is not sufficient to show that the new medical intervention actually works as claimed. The question must also be asked: Is the new medical intervention cost-effective? The previous chapter discussed this question in terms of cost limits. But in order to estimate the true cost of a medical intervention, it is essential to have an accurate picture of its efficacy. If, for example, the number of deaths prevented by a screening procedure for early detection of cancer is actually less than claimed, then the real cost (dollars per QALY) will be correspondingly higher.

Ideally, research studies should include an estimate of the real cost of any proposed new treatment. This need not necessarily be done with each and every RCT. After all, this is probably too complex for most clinical investigators. But before things go too far and people are demanding large-scale funding for population-wide implementation of the new procedure, with promises of the many lives to be saved, then a serious assessment of cost-effectiveness is essential. But to make this credible it is essential that cost-effectiveness studies be written in such a manner that a non-expert can understand them and be in a position to question some of the assumptions and calculations. They should also not be written by authors who have a conflict of interest, such as financial ties with the industry in question. Alas, studies that use cost-effectiveness "models" are seldom written in a transparent manner and few of them disclose any possible conflicts of interests of the authors.

Unfortunately, commercial interests pose a major obstacle against proper implementation of the above suggestions. We routinely find that they give much more priority to presenting their product in a way that encourages sales rather than to presenting a full and honest picture. And these biases commonly enter into published studies found in the medical literature. This subject is explored in the following chapter.

References

1 Rothman KJ, Michels KB (1994) The continuing unethical use of placebo controls. *N Engl J Med.* **331**: 394–8.
2 World Medical Association (2004). Available from www.wma.net/e/policy/63.htm (accessed 23 November 2005).
3 Furukawa TA, Guyatt GH, Griffith LE (2002) Can we individualize the "number needed to treat?" An empirical study of summary effect measures in meta-analyses. *Int J Epidemiol.* **31**: 72–6.

Chapter 3

Conflict of interest: a major problem in medical research

Joy Fraser

Introduction

Medical research is based on the public's trust that the interests of the subjects and of the public good will take priority over other interests. However, there is a serious danger that conflicts of interest (COIs) will lead to bias in research in various ways that threaten the integrity of the research process; this is of particular concern in drug trials.[1] This danger has become more acute in recent decades as major commercial corporate interests have steadily come to exert a major influence on research in our universities.

COIs may, and often will, arise when the obligations of the investigator to the research subjects and to the public good are influenced or biased by the interests of others, especially by the interests of the research sponsors or of the investigators. These interests could include the financial interests of the research sponsor, benefits of various types for the researchers (such as financial gain, job security, or promotion), or institutional goals.[2]

If bias is introduced it can affect any stage of a clinical study, including its design, the types of subjects selected for the study, the degree and veracity of the information participants receive about the risks and potential harms, the collection of the data itself, and in the reporting and publication (or nonpublication) of the research results.[2] Because physicians make life and death decisions based on published research, bias at any stage of the research process in biomedical research can have serious effects on human health. It also has major cost implications in that the financial motives of companies can lead to increased sales of highly priced medical products when perfectly adequate, but much cheaper ones, are available.

In this chapter I describe how medical COIs develop, the consequences they may have on the results of medical research, and how this can erode public trust in the medical system. For the most part I will focus on clinical trials on drugs and how their conduct has led to uncertainty about the safety, value, and effectiveness of drugs and devices that go to market.

The case of David Healy graphically illustrates the dangers of COIs. In 2001 he accepted a position as clinical director of the mood and anxiety disorders program at the Centre for Addictions and Mental Health and as professor of psychiatry at the University of Toronto. But before starting in his new position he was de-hired after giving a lecture about the danger that some of the most widely prescribed antidepressants, such as Prozac®, can lead to suicide in some types of patients. Healy expressed his opinion that despite the controversy over Prozac and other selective serotonin reuptake inhibitors (SSRIs), no research had been undertaken to examine risk factors. He estimated that a quarter of a million people had attempted to commit suicide because of Prozac and 25 000 had succeeded.[3]

After Healy's lecture, University of Toronto officials apparently asked the opinion of Charles Nemeroff, a professor of pharmacology at Emory University in Atlanta, Georgia. He happened to be at Healy's presentation and has links and shareholdings with Eli Lily, GlaxoSmithKline (GSK), and Pfizer, the three companies which make SSRIs. According to the news reports, Nemeroff had been openly hostile toward Healy and subsequently berated him from conducting research on the effects of SSRIs.[3–6] Ironically, it emerged in 2004 that GSK had conducted a trial during the 1990s which showed that their SSRI drug (paroxetine; known as Paxil® in North America and Seroxat® in the UK) may increase the risk of suicide, supporting what Healy had been saying several years earlier.[7,8] In 1998 GSK wrote an internal memo saying that it would be ''commercially unacceptable'' to admit that the drug was ineffective for depression in teenagers. The unreliability of published studies on SSRIs is discussed later in the chapter.

The lesson that emerges from this chapter is that big pharmaceutical companies have their own golden rule: He who has the gold makes the rules.

The stages of research

The most effective means medical science has come up with to determine the effectiveness of a drug or other treatment is to conduct randomized, controlled, double-blind clinical trials (RCTs). This research tool was described in Chapter 2. But before a clinical trial can even be planned, major steps in the research process must be carried out, and this is one area where COIs can have a major impact. For the purpose of this chapter I will mostly use drug therapy to illustrate the problem. However, the methods for testing some other types of therapy, radiation treatment for example, are similar.

According to Bero and Rennie:[9]

> The ''ideal'' published drug study ... would assess the effectiveness, toxicity, convenience, and cost of a new drug compared with available alternatives, would be designed to reduce systematic bias; and would draw conclusions that flow directly from the results. Such an ideal study would be conducted in an unbiased and ethical manner, and there would be evidence that measures were taken to ensure the quality of the data. The results of the ideal drug study would be published, regardless of study outcome. When published, the drug study would have been peer-reviewed and independent of sponsor influences.

Let us see how closely the real world conforms to this ideal.

Learning about the nature of a particular disease or condition is the first and most time-consuming step in the process of researching and developing drugs and biomedical products. Basic research about the details of how a disease comes about, and possible means to treat or cure it, is usually conducted in noncommercial laboratories, such as those in universities. Funding for this phase usually comes, at least in part, from the government. Subsequently, investigators set out to find or create a drug that will safely and effectively interfere with the chain of events causing the disease. Of the many substances with the potential to exploit as drugs, only a few pass the preclinical stage and go on to be tested in humans. During her 20 years as editor of the *New England Journal of Medicine* Angell[10] had a front-row seat when it came to the influence of the drug industry on medical research. She suggested that the most difficult and one of the most costly phases of the research and development process is this front-end part and it is often not funded by commercial enterprises.

Once a possible drug has been identified, it is then tested on animals to study its pharmacologic and toxic effects. This is often initiated and funded by a pharmaceutical company. If the initial results show promise, the drug company will seek approval to begin testing in humans. Before doing so, the company is required to submit a protocol for clinical trials to federal agencies and, subsequently, to institutional review boards. Clinical testing of drugs in humans is regulated by federal agencies, such as the Food and Drug Administration (FDA) in the USA. If research is funded by federal agencies (for example, the National Institutes of Health [NIH] in the USA), the protocol must be approved through other ethical approval bodies as well, so as to ensure the protection of human subjects. Unfortunately, as we shall see, this approval process has led to inadequate protection of human subjects.

Upon approval of the drug protocol, clinical investigators conduct small studies, first on small numbers of healthy volunteers and then on actual patients. If the drug survives this stage of testing, then the investigators proceed to an RCT, known as a Phase III study, in order to evaluate the safety and efficacy of the drug in larger numbers of patients. Finally, there are Phase IV studies where drugs that are already on the market are tested to find new uses for them to expand the market.

Conflicts of interest in approval, funding, and government regulators

In Canada, receipt of federal research funds from one or more of the agencies of the Tri-Council for research involving humans is contingent upon compliance with research ethics guidelines.[11]

When it comes to clinical trials for testing and marketing drugs, all Canadian researchers are required by Health Canada regulations to follow the International Convention on Harmonization of Good Clinical Practice. However, there have been recent concerns expressed about COIs within the councils responsible for establishing and administering the policies for ethical research in human subjects. There is a major conflict within the research councils between their primary role as promoters of research, including advancing industrial and social objectives, and their secondary role of protecting research subjects.[11] The ethics side of the job is the responsibility of the Panel on Research Ethics, which develops, interprets, and implements the Tri-Council Policy Statement (TCPS). However, its members are appointed by and report to the presidents of the three Canadian research agencies that represent social science, humanities, and science and industry. This therefore creates a difficult challenge for the research councils: to balance the objectives of promoting research with that of protecting human subjects. In fact, in November 2002 the Standing Committee on Ethics of the Canadian Institutes of Health Research (CIHR) unanimously endorsed a motion that: "There is a systemic conflict of interest in the dual role of the federal funding councils ... to both promote research and regulate its ethical conduct."[12]

A similar situation prevails in the USA. Campbell *et al.*[13] noted that while government agencies have policies and practices to protect against COIs in biomedical and health-related sciences, they are confusing and inconsistently applied. These authors describe difficulties in uncovering accurate information about government–industry relationships and highlight concerns released in the popular press about "lucrative financial arrangements between senior scientists at the NIH and industry which resulted in questions from congress about the nature and extent of these arrangements." Apparently, consulting relationships between 1995 and 2004 increased between NIH scientists and industry to the extent that some senior officials received from tens of thousands to over a hundred thousand dollars. In fact, Campbell *et al.*[13] observed that these consulting relationships "existed with companies that stood to benefit financially from the actions of the NIH officials. Such relationships have the potential to color objectivity in the grant-making process and to undermine the credibility of NIH."

The problem of systemic COI in the agencies that fund and regulate medical research continues in one form or another throughout the entire medical research process. Indeed, this has come under intense scrutiny by both the lay and professional press. Health Action International[14] berated the influence of the drug industry on government regulators, and voiced objections to the fact that the latter are funded by the very products of the industries they are assessing. They maintain that the corruption of regulators and their reluctance to challenge the drug industry is well illustrated by their failure to address the dangers associated with Vioxx® in the USA and Seroxat in the UK. The problems with these drugs are discussed in the following chapter.

Conflicts of interest in subject selection

Drug companies need to find subjects as quickly as possible so they can test the drugs, get them to market, and make a profit. In their quest for human guinea-pigs, they often rely on doctors to recruit patients. Alternately, subjects may be procured through means such as advertisements in the media. Another means used increasingly by pharmaceutical companies is to subcontract the task to contract research organizations (CRO).[10] A thousand or so CROs operating around the world establish networks of physicians with whom they collaborate. The physicians who recruit patients for clinical trials or administer study drugs and monitor their effects are paid well. CROs, with their revenues of billions of dollars from the drug companies, can offer doctors huge sums. In the USA, this amounted to an average of $7000 per patient in 2001. In addition, physicians are sometimes paid "bonuses for rapid enrollment ... up to $12 000 for each patient enrolled, plus another $30 000 on the enrollment of the sixth patient."[10]

This lucrative business has attracted media attention. CanWest News Service had discovered, as part of an investigation into clinical research, that private research companies had been going through confidential medical records, searching for people with medical conditions like arthritis, depression, and diabetes. Such practice is a violation of federal privacy laws.[15] Their investigation uncovered that these research companies were "pressuring Canadian doctors to enroll patients quickly into trials, engaging in questionable recruiting practices and are at times conducting trials that are not ethically or scientifically sound."[15] According to this news report, Dr Kam Shojania, a physician who was heading clinical trials at an arthritis research center in Vancouver, stated that companies pay CAN$3000–$5000 for every patient he enrolls. One trial paid CAN$18 000 per patient. Moreover, he claimed he was frequently pressured by research promoters wanting to set up more trials, because, as the journalist observed, "Shojania has ready access to something they cannot buy: human volunteers." The amount spent on clinical trials each year in Canada is estimated to be between $800 million and $1 billion, so it is easy to see why huge sums are available for recruitment of subjects.

Morin and colleagues[16] observed that nonmonetary incentives to physicians can also be used to encourage the timely recruitment of subjects. These might include offers from drug companies to provide lab equipment, more research contracts, and invitations to meetings in interesting parts of the world. This can lead to the problem of role-conflict that occurs when the research scientist is also the clinical practitioner. Researchers seek new findings with the hope that therapeutic benefits will be revealed, whereas the practitioners' focus is (or should be) on the well-being of their patients.

Munro[15] discussed some of the common problems that occur in the hundreds of research projects being conducted in Canada: trials were not properly approved; some where data that might have harmed the sale of drugs were suppressed; deals signed between drug companies, doctors, and universities were kept secret; where investigators failed to report serious adverse reactions; and where researchers failed to warn patients of the dangers and side effects associated with drug trials and medical experiments. Munro also pointed out that although doctors get paid hefty fees to recruit, they do not declare this to patients involved in the studies and there is no guarantee the studies will be completed or that the data collected will ever be released, even though patients and doctors are often told that their participation in trials will lead to new knowledge. But, more importantly, financial and other incentives can compromise physicians' judgments when enrolling subjects in trials. Munro also noted that while there is detailed information about how many animals are used in Canadian research studies each year, no one knows exactly how many humans are used in clinical trials.

Reinforcing this concern DuVal[17] argued that if investigators have a "financial interest in success of the research, such as equity interest in the sponsor, or if the researcher has come to rely upon the sponsor for research funding or for personal income, the researcher has financial interests in adequate recruitment and positive results." He pointed out that researchers and institutions may own shares, options, or other interests in biotechnology companies formed for the purposes of "exploiting research findings," and this could cause the researcher to "recruit subjects inappropriately, to downplay risks and exaggerate benefits, to cut corners on exclusion/inclusion criteria, or to underreport adverse events." Therefore, pharmaceutical companies may be able to supply financial resources and their drug to academic researchers who have access to patients, but ethical problems are aggravated in such situations.[18]

Angell[10] also suggested that one risk of paying doctors to recruit subjects is that this may lead to patients being enrolled who are not really eligible. She speculates that, "If it means an extra $30 000 for you to enroll a patient in an asthma study, you might very well be tempted to say your next patient has asthma whether he does or not." It is reasonable to believe that the conflict between the two hats that doctors wear – physician and investigator – could lead to the investigator circumventing study enrollment criteria or bypassing established random selection processes. In addition, a bias can be introduced by selecting patients that have a greater probability of reacting positively to the drug. Bodenheimer[19] suggested that by selecting patients who are younger and healthier and with milder manifestations of the disease, the drug being studied will likely appear to be more effective and show fewer side effects than might be the case in the actual target population.

The concern about bias in the selection of patients has also been expressed by Rochon et al.,[20] who opposed the "lack of inclusion and representation of target populations," noting that in major trials of nonsteroidal anti-inflammatory drugs (NSAIDs) only 2.1% of the participants were 65 years or older, even though the largest users of these drugs and those who are likely to have more serious side effects are the elderly. Bero and Rennie[9] emphasized that in the past, women, the elderly, and ethnic groups were excluded from studies of drugs that were later widely used by these groups. This is an important point because drug metabolism, and hence effectiveness and safety, differ in different groups, and yet data on effectiveness and toxicity are often not available. This poses potentially serious risks for patients.

Conflicts of interest in informing subjects of risks

Regulatory bodies, as well as institutional research ethics boards, have been set up for the purpose of protecting human research subjects. An essential ingredient of the process is informed consent. This means that investigators must explain to potential participants the nature of the study and its risks and benefits. Participants must also be assured that they are free to refuse to participate and may withdraw at any time during the study without negative consequences. The participants must also be told that their confidentiality will be protected, who will have access to personal information collected, and how the data will be used. A more recent requirement, and one that is central to this chapter, is the requirement for investigators to inform participants about the possibility of commercialization of the research findings. Participants must also be fully informed about COIs, potential or real, that may be present among the researchers, their institutions, or the research sponsors. They must also be informed about how the research will be published and how participants will be informed of the study results.[12] And yet, despite the proliferation of organizations, policies, and guidelines which have been established to prevent unethical behavior in medical research, Schuppli and McDonald[11] maintain that there are still serious concerns about protection of participants. Some of the evidence was given above.

Even when consent is obtained, the veracity of this consent can be questioned when subjects are unduly influenced by their relationship with the researcher. For example, patients might be influenced because they trust their doctor or believe that they will be cured by the drug being studied; these factors may cloud their judgment and ability to assess the advantages and disadvantages of participating in the clinical trial. The physician "may not be inclined to emphasize how the experimental treatment differs from the care that is ordinarily provided, the additional risks involved, or the lack of direct benefit to the participant." Munro[15] described a recent study comparing treatments for acute respiratory distress syndrome funded by the NIH and conducted in one Canadian and over 12 American medical centers. The patients, many so ill they were heavily sedated and on ventilators in intensive care, were asked to participate in experiments that involved changing lung pressures and fluid therapy so that investigators could determine which techniques had higher or lower death rates. After an investigation, the US Office for Human Research Protections reprimanded the centers for failing to adequately assess the risks and benefits to patients and for failing to ensure that the "highly vulnerable" patients and their legal guardians were properly informed of the possibility of a higher risk of death.

When clinical trials are conducted with patients afflicted with terminal illnesses, they are particularly vulnerable. The patients and their families' perception of the risks and benefits can be severely distorted in their desperate search for a cure.

Clearly, the rights and interest of patients are not being served if they are not fully informed of the risks, nor is the public good or medical science being served by the suppression of adverse drug reactions and other negative results. Health Action International[14] believes the corruption of medicine has resulted in a system where the science is no longer the driver of the development and production of drugs, and public safety has become a secondary issue. The public "do not and cannot know if every time they take a pill or participate in a research trial, they are endangering their lives, because every level of medicine's production system has been corrupted."

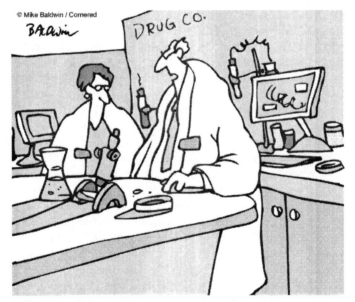

"Do a double-blind test. Give the new drug to rich patients and a placebo to the poor. No sense getting their hopes up. They couldn't afford it even if it works."

Bias in study design

Drug companies tend to put their efforts into developing drugs with the largest market, such as drugs for arthritis and high blood pressure. Capturing the market share and making a profit is their driving force, and product competition is a key element of research carried out by the pharmaceutical industry. Bolaria and Dickenson[21] noted that, "Instead of developing drugs with the greatest health potential, the companies generally direct their research efforts towards developing drugs with the greatest profit potential."

Angell[10] commented that one of the problems in the ties connecting medicine and biomedical researchers to industry is that researchers may choose topics on the basis of whether they can obtain industry funding rather than because the studies are important. This, in turn, means that research on drugs and devices increases, while research on the causes of disease declines. In addition, she predicted that research will be skewed in order to find insignificant differences between drugs, and that those differences will be exploited to get the drugs to market. Because drug companies make more profit from new drugs, which they can patent, rather than from old ones, it is not surprising that they mainly fund studies that demonstrate the effectiveness of new drugs. Indeed, pharmaceutical companies fund almost all research on new drugs.

Drug companies typically test new drugs against placebos because this maximizes the chance that the new drug will appear effective. If the control group were given an existing drug, this might reveal that the new drug is, in reality, no better, or even inferior, to the existing drug. In Canada, however, under the Tri-Council policy, it is not acceptable to use placebos as controls in clinical trials except in certain circumstances.[22] Examples include treatment of minor conditions, where there is no standard treatment, where the therapeutic advantage of the standard treatment is questionable, or where the cost or limited supply of an existing effective treatment makes it prohibitive.

Funding and publication of research results

In a study of the scope and impact of financial COIs in biomedical research, Bekelman et al.[23] found that between 23% and 28% of researchers have industry affiliations, and roughly two-thirds of academic institutions hold equity in start-up companies that sponsor research undertaken in those institutions. This demonstrates how, in addition to benefiting from research funds, physicians and researchers often benefit financially when drugs are approved for market and the drug companies make a profit. The various forms of COI resulting from academia–industry ties frequently lead to misleading or even false outcomes of drug studies. There is strong evidence to substantiate that this indeed is what is routinely happening. This seems to be a case of "He who pays the piper calls the tune."

Several carefully researched studies have reported that when studies of new drugs are funded by drug companies, the results are more likely to favor the new drug than when funding is received from other sources. Bhandari et al.[24] examined the results of 332 RCTs published between 1999 and 2001 in eight leading surgical and five medical journals. Industry funding was declared in 122 (37%) of the trials. In both surgical and medical trials that funding was associated with statistically significant results in favor of the new industry product. Adding to this evidence, Lexchin and colleagues[25] conducted a meta-analysis of research articles published between 1966 and 2002, and found systematic bias in the outcomes of research funded by pharmaceutical companies. They found clear evidence that studies sponsored by drug companies were more likely to have positive outcomes favoring the product made by the sponsor. This was shown across a wide range of diseases, different drugs and drug classes, and all types of research. Similarly, Bekelman et al.[23] examined 1140 published studies and concluded that industry-sponsored studies were 3.6 times more likely to reach pro-industry conclusions than non-industry studies.

Perlis and colleagues[26] carried out an analysis of RCTs published in four major dermatology journals from 2000 to 2003. All four journals require authors to report funding sources and potential COIs. Of 179 RCTs, 102 (57%) reported industry support, while 47 (26%) did not identify funding sources. At least one author in 77 (43%) of the studies reported a potential financial COI: 70 (39%) included at least one author who was also employed by the sponsor, three (2%) included stock-holders in the industry sponsors, and 33 (18%) had at least one author who had received consulting fees, speaker's fees, or other sponsor support. Studies that were industry-sponsored and employee-authored were more likely (65% vs 35%) to report positive findings than studies that were not industry sponsored. In many of the studies important information relating to COIs was missing and in each such case the authors treated the report as if there were no COIs. For this reason the study probably underestimated the association between industry support and the reporting of positive findings.

Melander et al.[27] reviewed 42 RCTs sponsored by drug companies in order to investigate the impact of publication bias. The focus was on five SSRIs, a class of antidepressants, such as Prozac, that were discussed at the beginning of this chapter with respect to the David Healy scandal. Over half of the studies contributed to two or more publications each, significant effects of drugs were published more often than studies with nonsignificant results, and many publications ignored negative results and reported favorable analysis only. These investigators concluded that due to this evidence of duplicate publication, selective publication, and selective reporting, any attempt to recommend specific SSRIs for major depression based on the published data is likely to be based on biased results.

How do drug companies manage to transform their funding for RCTs into such high levels of "success" in the published studies reporting results? They can engineer this in several different ways. Inappropriate study design, which was discussed earlier, is one way. Another tactic is publication bias: the selective publication of results. Studies that produce results that do not support the sponsors' drugs are less likely to be published. This problem is exemplified by the Celebrex® fiasco. Schafer[28] described how, although the full data set was available, only partial results of the clinical trial for Celebrex were published. These results, based on six months of data, indicated that the drug causes lower rates of stomach and intestinal ulcers than two existing drugs used for treating arthritis. Following publication Celebrex became a "blockbuster" drug. But subsequently, the full year of data became available and this revealed that Celebrex is no safer than existing arthritis drugs. The fact that eight of the study's authors were paid medical consultants for Pharmacia, which funded the study, and the other eight were company employees, underscores the problem with COI and issues related to objectivity. Problems associated with this drug are further discussed in Chapter 7.

Drug companies have been known to use heavy-handed techniques, such as bullying and legal enforcement of restrictive clauses in contracts, in order to suppress negative findings. This is clearly demonstrated in the case described by Rennie[29] where a drug company blocked, for seven years, the publication of a study of Synthroid by Dong and colleagues that had results unfavorable to the drug company, Boots Pharmaceuticals. Rennie remarked: "It is hard to believe that the sponsors would have made such extraordinary efforts to delay and block publication of the study for such a very long time and for such an extraordinary number of specious reasons if the results had shown Synthyroid to be better [than other preparations of levothyroxine]."

Hailey[30] wrote about the litigious means that industry sometimes uses to dispute research findings and block the dissemination of negative results. Ritter[31] described how corporate ties can infringe on academic freedom when he cites the case of James Kahn, a researcher in San Francisco at the University of California, who was doing research on a promising HIV vaccine. Kahn's research was supported by the drug's manufacturer, Immune Response Corporation, which had signed a contract with the university, for clinical testing of its product produced under the trade name Remune. When Kahn discovered that the drug did not work and attempted to publish his findings, Immune Response pressured him to alter his data to make the results look more favorable. Upon his refusal, the company sued him on the grounds that release of negative results would disclose proprietary information. When Kahn proceeded to publish, the company published its own clinical data to refute his findings. Ritter suggested that the case illustrated that: "The ethics of business and the ethics of science mix like gasoline and water."[31]

This view is echoed by Lewis et al.,[32] who highlighted the intimidating tactics used by the pharmaceutical industry against researchers in Canadian cases involving "Bristol-Myers Squibb lawsuit against the Canadian Coordinating Office on Health Technology Assessment (CCOHTA) to suppress its statin report, and the AstraZeneca legal threat against Anne Holbrook for her review of medications for stomach ulcers." Bullying techniques were also used by a pharmaceutical company in the case of Nancy Olivieri at the University of Toronto. At the time she was a specialist conducting a RCT of an experimental iron-chelation drug for the treatment of thalassemia.[33] Her case is a prime example of what can happen when clinical investigators unwittingly sign contracts that protect the interests of the sponsor but not the public or the safety of participants in drug trials. The investigator, Olivieri, attempted to meet her legal and ethical responsibilities to inform participants of unexpected risks. Apotex, the sponsor, asserted their contractual right, through a confidentiality clause, to control the communication of information, including risks, and to terminate the trial without prior notice. Apotex disputed Olivieri's findings and attempted to block her efforts to inform patients of the risks.

In addition to nonpublication of results from RCTs, a lesser problem is delayed publication. Blumenthal et al.[34] found that 20% of 2167 life sciences faculty in 50 American universities reported delays of over six months in the publication of research results, and 28% said this was due to "slow dissemination of undesired results to allow time to negotiate a patent, or to settle disputes over the ownership of intellectual property."

The next step after RCTs have been published is the review and interpretation of their meaning. And here, too, we see a close association between COIs and the stated opinions of the experts. Stelfox et al.[35] reviewed 70 reports in order to examine the links between doctors' published support of the use of calcium channel antagonists to treat high blood pressure and their financial relationship with drug manufacturers. They found that among the authors who supported the use of this class of drugs, all but one (96%) had received funding from the drug manufacturers, whereas, conversely, those who criticized their safety were much less likely (43%) to have financial ties.

The same story emerges when we look at clinical practice guidelines (CPG). Choudhry and colleagues[36] investigated the extent and nature of interactions between drug companies and authors of CPG. They compared the financial incentives the authors received from the pharmaceutical industry and the amount of interaction they disclosed in the published guidelines. Of the 82 authors who responded to their survey (83% response rate), 87% had some form of interaction with the pharmaceutical industry, with 58% receiving financial support for research and 38% serving as employees or consultants to drug firms. Most of them had relationships with five or six different drug companies. All of the CPG for seven of the 10 disease states included in the study had at least one author who had a relationship with the drug industry, and 59% of these authors had relationships with companies whose products were included in the guidelines they wrote. Furthermore, although almost half of the CPG authors reported that their relationship with the drug industry was discussed prior to developing the guidelines, in only one of the 44 published guidelines included in the study did the authors declare they had a financial relationship with the drug company and none declared any potential COI. The extent of COIs among the authors of CPG was confirmed in a larger survey carried out by the journal *Nature*.[37] The investigators looked at 200 CPG from around the world. One alarming finding was that 49% of the CPG did not include any details as to the COIs of authors.

Consistent with the various findings described above, Blumenthal et al.,[34,38] Bodenheimer,[19] and Love[39] have documented the following: medical scientists report delayed publications of their results for over six months for commercial reasons; published findings in journals and findings of studies presented at scientific meetings are nearly always favorable to the study drug when the study is funded by the drug manufacturer; and study drugs are given more favorable reviews when authors have financial ties to industry sponsors.

The problem of COIs causing distortions in published reports may reach into the actual medical journals. Glassman et al.[40] evaluated six nonprofit medical organizations in an effort to quantify potential COIs for professional medical societies stemming from advertising revenues generated from the pharmaceutical industry. One primary clinical journal was evaluated from each of the parent organizations of the following societies: the American College of Cardiology; the American College of Physicians; the American Medical Association; the American Thoracic Society; the Infectious Diseases Society of America; and the Massachusetts Medical Society. They calculated the income from drug advertisements in journals as a percentage of total income of the corresponding society. While there was substantial variation, they estimated the six journals raised $46 million from pharmaceutical advertising in 1996, with five out of six obtaining over 10% of their total revenue from advertising in a single journal. Pharmaceutical advertisements generated as much or nearly as much revenue for four of the six organizations as did membership dues and other fees. In the case of the Massachusetts Medical Society, advertising revenue from the *New England Journal of Medicine* provided 21% of its income and was over eight times more than the amount received from member contributions. The study authors concluded that pharmaceutical advertising revenues in journals can lead to potential COIs.

Academia–medicine–industry partnerships: viewpoints

The cases documented in this chapter reveal a system-wide problem related to corporate sponsorship in the whole research and publication process. The essence of academic integrity and the fundamental goal of medical research to advance scientific knowledge are compromised. Medical researchers may be pressured to suppress research results that are not consistent with the financial interests of pharmaceutical companies. As a result, without rigorous and objective testing, useless and even harmful drugs are being developed and marketed. Physicians who are perusing the literature in order to make informed decisions about what to prescribe gain a distorted picture of the merits of various drugs, including their clinical effectiveness, adverse effects, convenience, and cost. A predictable result of this is that doctors will change their prescribing habits in directions that serve the profits of the drug industry rather than either the health of their patients or the budgets of those who must pay for the drugs.[41] The tax relief given to this for-profit research takes millions of dollars of public money away from potentially better uses, such as research conducted by independent and unbiased researchers. In brief, sponsorship bias and COI in medical research has serious consequences – it kills people and leads to huge waste of money.

Alas, the response by large numbers of academic institutions, journals, and other organizations with a legitimate interest in this problem has been seriously inadequate. McCrary *et al.*[42] conducted a national survey of 297 American institutions to analyze their policies on disclosure of COIs in biomedical research. Their study included 127 medical schools, 170 other research institutions, 48 journals in basic science and clinical medicine, and 17 federal agencies. They reported that 6% of the 250 institutions (84% response rate) had no policies on COI. Of those that did, there was significant variability among the policies. Less than half of the journals (43%) had policies requiring disclosure of COI and all but one of the federal agencies relied on institutional discretion, with only four having explicit policies addressing COI. Similarly, Lo *et al.*,[43] in their study at 10 American medical schools concerning clinical trials, found that current COI policies vary widely and have substantial shortcomings.

How did medical science end up so dependent on and manipulated by industry? There are several reasons offered in the literature about why this relationship between academic medicine and industry has developed. According to Angell[44] one commonly used justification for these extensive ties is that academic institutions need the money. Cuts in government funding have certainly left academic institutions looking for research funding, and when industry saw an opportunity to profit from university research, they were quick to step in. Angell notes that the Bayh–Dole Act is frequently used to justify academia–industry partnerships, with the view that such ties are necessary to ensure technology transfer and that clinical medicine benefits from more contact between the two.

In the USA, before the passage of the Bayh–Dole Act, there was a perception that federally funded research belonged in the public domain. However, this research rarely led to viable products or services. According to Henderson and Smith[45] "prior to the Act's passage, the federal government held title to roughly 28 000 patents, only 5% of which were licensed to industry for commercial development." These authors argued that the Bayh–Dole Act created an "implied duty for government grantees/contractors, including academic medical institutions, to commercialize subject interventions, and implicitly encouraged academia–industry collaboration in this pursuit." They suggest that universities and the public have benefited greatly from the act through technology transfer activities which created jobs, economic activity, useful products, and, in the case of patient care, medical products and healthcare technologies that might not have reached the clinical applications stage.

Bodenheimer,[19] Ioannidis,[46] Parks and Disis,[47] DuVal,[17] and others have identified both benefits and COIs when industry partners are involved in biomedical research. Similarly, Harmon and Sherwal[6] observed: "Enhanced university–industry links have provided avenues for academics to be more involved in R&D, attracted substantial additional financial resources for universities, provided important financial support and career opportunities for PhD students and stimulated major expansion in technology transfer and research commercialization."

Lieberwitz[48] described the change in relationship between universities and private financial supporters as a "shift from corporate contribution to corporate investment in academia." He argued that the commercialization of academic research may well reduce both the scope and quality of the research. "The growth of university practices modeled on for-profit businesses, including priorities on commercially viable research, protection of private ownership rights of intellectual property, and increases in secrecy, undermines the communal academic culture that encourages innovation and experimentation." He maintains that defining the public interest as synonymous with the corporate interest ignores both the COIs between the public interest and private corporate interests, and fails to acknowledge the resulting damage to the public interest from privatization and commercialization of academic research. The pursuit of commercialization does not normally exist within the mission of the university, which has focused on education, research, and, in the case of health professions such as medicine, patient care. Hence, there have been many criticisms and concerns about industry involvement in academia and their conflicting interests. It is widely understood that industry is governed by a business ethic, operating within a competitive environment, motivated by profits, and responsible to investors and shareholders, whereas academic institutions are governed by a professional ethic, operating in a collegial environment, motivated by the quest for truth and knowledge, and responsible to the public as a whole.[45] In fact, many have come to believe that the influence of the pharmaceutical industry has lead to dishonesty and corruption.

Gotzsche[49] also challenged the reliance on industry funding arguing:

> It is clear that governments could save money and treat patients better by investing much more in trials and academic trial centres than by relying on industry's own trials and conclusions. Who would buy a washing machine that is five or 10 times more expensive than other machines just because its manufacturer

has compared it with other machines and claims that it is the best? Unfortunately, such absurdities are often seen in health care, and are allowed to happen even in the absence of any direct head-to-head comparisons.

The literature is replete with concerns about the tenuous relationship between academia, medicine, and industry. The disparities, the tensions, and the potential risks inherent in this relationship are reflected in the works of Krimsky,[50] Feldman and Desrochers,[51] and others. Campbell *et al.*[13] noted that "several empirical studies have supported the existence of risks associated with secrecy in science, bias in the reporting of research, negative side effects on education and conflicts of interest." Sackett and Oxman[52] called the relationship between medicine and the drug industry "an amalgamation of the world's two oldest professions," implying that medicine has sold itself to industry by using an array of strategies to make sure they protect industries' "worthless product as [they] shepherd it through the minefields sewn by objective scientists, fussy ethics committees, conscientious journal editors, writers of evidence based guidelines, and licensing bodies." Schafer[53] agrees that the relationship between medicine and industry is ethically problematic because every corporate gift or grant to medical students, physicians, researchers, hospitals, and universities comes with strings attached and puts the recipient in a COI situation. Doctors "have a fiduciary duty to their patients – a duty to put the patient's interest first – but they now have another interest, a 'vested interest' in the success of the new drug being tested."

References

1   Holmes DR, Firth BG, James A *et al.* (2004) Results of expert meetings. Conflict of interest. *Am Heart J.* **147**: 228–37.
2   Canadian Institutes of Health Research, Natural Sciences and Engineering Research Council of Canada, Social Sciences and Humanities Research Council of Canada (1998) Tri-Council Policy Statement: Ethical Conduct for Research Involving Humans, 1998 (with 2000, 2002, and 2005 amendments). Available from: www.pre.ethics.gc.ca/english/policystatement/policystatement.cfm (accessed November 23, 2005).
3   Boseley S (2001) Bitter pill. *Guardian*, May 7. Available from http://education.guardian.co.uk/businessofresearch/comment/0,,487530,00.html (accessed November 23, 2005).
4   CAUT Bulletin (2001) Academic freedom in jeopardy at Toronto. *CAUT Bulletin.* **48**: A1.
5   Angell M (2000) Is academic medicine for sale? *N Engl J Med.* **342**: 1516–8.
6   Harmon G, Sherwell V (2002) Risks in university–industry research links and the implications for university management. *Journal of Higher Education Policy Management.* **24**: 37–51.
7   Dyer O (2004) GlaxoSmithKline faces US lawsuit over concealment of trial results. *BMJ.* **328**: 1395.
8   Spurgeon D (2004) GlaxoSmithKline staff told not to publicise ineffectiveness of its drug. *BMJ.* **328**: 422.
9   Bero LA, Rennie D (1996) Influences on the quality of published drug studies. *Int J Technol Assess Health Care.* **12**: 209–37.
10 Angell M (2004) *The Truth about Drug Companies. How they Deceive Us and What to Do About It.* Random House, New York.
11 Schuppli CA, McDonald M (2005) Contrasting modes of governance for the protection of humans and animals in Canada: lessons for reform. *Health Law Review.* **13**: 97–107.
12 Canadian Institutes of Health Research Standing Committee on Ethics (2002) The Canadian Institutes of Health Research 3rd Meeting of the Standing Committee on Ethics, November 7. Available from www.cihr-irsc.gc.ca/e/16778.html (accessed November 23, 2005).
13 Campbell EG, Koski G, Zinner DE, Blumenthal D (2005) Managing the triple helix in the life sciences. *Issues Science Technology.* **21**: 48–52.

14 Health Action International (2004) *Attending to a Sick Industry*. A Health Action International Discussion Paper, 2004. Available from www.haiweb.org/pdf/sickindustry.pdf (accessed November 23, 2005).

15 Munro M (2004) Who is looking out for the human guinea pigs? Questionable recruitment practice enters grey zone. *Edmonton Journal*. February 23, A2.

16 Morin K, Rakatansky H, Riddick FA (2002) Managing conflicts of interest in the conduct of clinical trials. *JAMA* **287**: 78–84.

17 DuVal G (2005) The benefits and threats of research partnerships with industry. *Critical Care*. **9**: 309–10.

18 Bickford A (2004) Maintaining integrity in industry-sponsored research. American Medical Association, November. Available from www.ama-assn.org/ama/pub/category/13191.html (accessed November 23, 2005).

19 Bodenheimer T (2000) Uneasy alliance – clinical investigators and the pharmaceutical industry. *N Engl J Med*. **342**: 1539–44.

20 Rochon P, Berger PB, Cohen A *et al*. (1998) The evolution of clinical trials: inclusion and representation. *Can Med Assoc J*. **159**: 1373–4.

21 Bolaria SB, Dickenson HD (1994) *Health, Illness and Healthcare in Canada* (2e). Harcourt Brace, Toronto.

22 Interagency Advisory Panel on Research Ethics (2005) Tri-Council Policy Statement: Ethical Conduct for Research Involving Humans. Available from www.pre.ethics.gc.ca/english/policystatement/policystatement.cfm (accessed November 23, 2005).

23 Bekelman JE, Li Y, Gross GP (2003) Scope and impact of financial conflicts of interest in biomedical research: a systematic review. *JAMA*. **289**: 454–65.

24 Bhandari M, Busse JW, Jackowski D *et al*. (2004) Association between industry funding and statistically significant pro-industry findings in medical and surgical randomized trials. *Can Med Assoc J*. **170**: 477–80.

25 Lexchin J, Bero LA, Djulbegovic B, Clark O (2003) Pharmaceutical industry sponsorship and research outcome and quality: systematic review. *BMJ*. **326**: 1167–70.

26 Perlis CS, Harwood M, Perlis RH (2005) Extent and impact of industry sponsorship conflicts of interest in dermatology research. *J Am Acad Dermatol*. **52**: 967–71.

27 Melander H, Ahlqvist-Rastad J, Meijer G, Beermann B (2003) Evidence b(i)ased medicine-selective reporting from studies sponsored by pharmaceutical industry: review of studies in new drug applications. *BMJ*. **326**: 1171–3.

28 Schafer A (2003) Bad Rx – big pharma and medical research. *CAUT Bulletin*. October, A13.

29 Rennie D (1997) Thyroid storm. *JAMA*. **277**: 1238–43.

30 Hailey D (2000) Scientific harassment by pharmaceutical companies: time to stop. *Can Med Assoc J*. **162**: 212–3.

31 Ritter P (2001) City pages (Minneapolis/St Paul). July 4, 22. Available from http://citypages.com/databank/22/1074/article9665.asp?page=2 (accessed November 23, 2005).

32 Lewis S, Baird P, Evans RG *et al*. (2001) Dancing with the porcupine: rules for governing the university–industry relationship. *Can Med Assoc J*. **165**: 783–5.

33 Schafer A. (2004) Biomedical conflicts of interest: a defence of the sequestration thesis-learning from the cases of Nancy Olivieri and David Healy. *J Med Ethics*. **30**: 8–24.

34 Blumenthal D, Campbell EG, Anderson MS, Causino N, Louis KS (1997) Withholding research results in academic life science. Evidence from a national survey of faculty. *JAMA*. **277**: 1224–8.

35 Stelfox HT, Chua G, O'Rourke K, Detsky AS (1998) Conflict of interest in the debate over calcium-channel antagonists. *N Engl J Med*. **338**: 101–6.

36 Choudhry NK, Stelfox HT, Detsky AS (2002) Relationships between authors of clinical practice guidelines and the pharmaceutical industry. *JAMA*. **287**: 612–7.

37 Taylor R, Giles J (2005) Cash interests taint drug advice. *Nature*. **437**: 1070–1.

38 Blumenthal D, Causino N, Campbell EG, Louis KS (1996) Relationship between academic institutions and industry in the life sciences industry survey. *N Engl J Med*. **334**: 368–73.

39 Love J (2000) Where to draw the bottom line: financial conflict of interest in clinical research. *NIH Catalyst*. September–October. Available from http://lists.essential.org/pipermail/pharm-policy/2000-October/000377.html (accessed July 5, 2005).

40 Glassman PA, Hunter-Hayes J, Nakamura T (1999) Pharmaceutical advertising revenue and physician organizations: how much is too much? *West J Med*. **171**: 234–8.

41 Kassirer JP (2004) *On the Take: how medicine's complicity with big business can endanger your health*. Oxford University Press, Oxford.

42 McCrary SV, Anderson, CB, Jakovljevic J *et al.* (2000) A national survey of policies on disclosure of conflicts of interests in biomedical research. *N Engl J Med*. **343**: 1621–6.

43 Lo B, Wolf LE, Berkeley A (2000) Conflict-of-interest policies for investigators in clinical trials. *N Engl J Med*. **343**: 1616–20.

44 Angell M (2000) Is academic medicine for sale? *N Engl J Med*. **342**: 1516–8.

45 Henderson JA, Smith JJ (2000) Academia, Industry, and the Bayh–Dole Act: an implied duty to commercialize, 2002. Available from www.evptnrs.com/doleact.pdf (accessed November 23, 2005).

46 Ioannidis JP (2004) Materializing research promises: opportunities, priorities, and conflicts in translational medicine. *J Transl Med*. **2**: 5.

47 Parks MR, Disis ML (2004) Conflicts of interest in translational research. *J Transl Med*. **2**: 28. Available from http://.translational-medicine.com/content/2/1/28 (accessed August 22, 2005).

48 Lieberwitz RL (2005) Confronting the privatization and commercialization of academic research: an analysis of social implications at the local, national, and global levels. *Indiana J Global Legal Studies*. **12**: 109–52.

49 Gotzsche PC (2005) Research integrity and pharmaceutical industry sponsorship. *Med J Aust*. **182**: 549–50.

50 Krimsky S (2001) Journal policies on conflict of interest: if this is the therapy, what's the disease? *Psychother Psychosom*. **70**: 115–7.

51 Feldman MP, Desrochers P (2004) Truth for its own sake: academic culture and technology transfer at Johns Hopkins University. *Minerva*. **42**: 105–26.

52 Sackett DL, Oxman AD (2003) Harlot plc: an amalgamation of the world's two oldest professions. *BMJ*. **327**: 1442–5.

53 Schafer A (2002) Medicine, morals and money: dancing with porcupines or sleeping beside elephants? Available from www.umanitoba.ca/centres/ethics/articles/article2.html (accessed November 24, 2005).

Chapter 4

Drug regulation: two paradigms in conflict

Joel Lexchin

Introduction

Drug regulation would seem to be an easy task: make sure that the drugs that reach the public are safe and effective, and ensure that accurate information is provided about how to use these medications. In this view of things, espoused by consumer groups and public health activists, medications are seen as an essential element of the healthcare system and the regulatory authority exists to provide a service to the public. But the real world is not that simple. The vision of the purpose of regulation articulated in the opening sentence is not the only one. Another one, put forward by the pharmaceutical industry and its allies, holds that the main function is to facilitate industry's efforts to develop new products and to approve them as quickly as possible. In this view, medications are commodities and the regulatory authority exists to provide a service to the industry.

These visions are not completely polar opposites. Industry would agree that marketed medications should also be safe and effective, but it also is very clear that marketing authorization should not be held up by what it sees as undue delays in evaluating the trial data that it submits. To this end, in many countries drug companies fund part or all of the regulatory authority through user fees and, in return, expect timely approvals for their products. Companies also regard their data as proprietary and expect regulatory authorities to keep it confidential so as not to jeopardize their commercial activities. Consumer groups and health activists, on the other hand, concede that the drug companies are necessary to develop new products, but they are mainly focused on the quality of the products that emerge from the approval process, and are more interested in a thorough review than a rapid one. They also are generally in favor of transparency in the regulatory review process. Disease-focused groups sometimes differ from consumer groups on the question of the speed of drug approvals. While they still are concerned with safety, they often want what they see as new therapeutically important medications approved as quickly as possible.

The Food and Drug Administration (FDA)* in the USA is by far the largest and most influential regulatory authority in the world and this chapter will draw primarily on information about its functioning. In addition, examples from

---

*The FDA incorporates the Center for Drug Evaluation and Research (CDER), which regulates medicines derived through chemical synthesis, and the Center for Biologics Evaluation and Research (CBER), which regulates blood products, vaccines, and cellular/gene therapy.

Australia, Canada, the European Union (EU), New Zealand, and the UK will be explored so as to illustrate the competing visions of the agencies in these countries. A major focus will be on: the effects of the pharmaceutical industry on the process of approving new drugs; the level of postmarketing surveillance, transparency, and conflict of interest; and the control over promotion of drugs. In looking at these issues I will also emphasize how the two different models of drug regulation are expressed in the precautionary principle and risk management.

In brief, the precautionary principle holds that even in the absence of firm data showing that something is harmful, its approval should either be delayed or, if it is allowed on to the market, it should be under restricted conditions. Risk management, on the other hand, says that things should be assumed to be safe unless there is information to the contrary, and in general products should be allowed unfettered access to the market and once there largely left unattended. Risk management usually involves a risk–cost–benefit approach which has a "built-in bias in favor of technological benefits, which are immediate, highly predictable, and quantifiable (otherwise, the technology would have no market), and against the risk factors, which are discounted because they tend to be long term, less certain, and less easily quantified." While the precautionary principle is proactive in the sense that it assumes that "It is better to design and deploy the technologies in ways that prevent or avoid the potential harms, or guarantee the management of these risks within limits of acceptability, than to move ahead with them on the assumption that unanticipated harms can be ameliorated with future revisions or technological 'fixes'."[1]

Finally, after analyzing the regulatory systems I will look at possible reforms.

Historical perspectives on regulatory authorities

The various regulatory authorities arose out of particular historical situations. As Wiktorowicz[2] points out in her monograph on drug regulation in the USA, the pluralist model, with its laissez-faire approach to the participation of private interests in decision making, has predominated. European countries, with their centralized state authority, have favored a corporatist model with a pattern of orderly, tightly knit, state–society relationships that involves negotiations and accommodation with industry. In contrast, industry in the USA does not directly participate in the running of the FDA, but has an indirect influence on decisions through its ability to challenge them in the courts. Moreover, the US system is characterized by a high level of political oversight. Finally, the Canadian Therapeutic Products Directorate (TPD),* although better resourced than its European equivalents, is relatively less well resourced than the FDA and as a result operates through a system known as "clientele pluralism."[3] In such a system the state has a high degree of concentration of power in one agency, the TPD, but a low degree of autonomy. In Canada, government regulation of drug safety, quality, and efficacy is almost solely the responsibility of the TPD. But the state does not possess the

---

*The TPD is part of Health Canada. It is the equivalent of the CDER, while the Biologics and Genetic Therapies Directorate is the equivalent of the CBER, which regulates blood products, vaccines, and cellular/gene therapy.

wherewithal to undertake the elaborate clinical and preclinical trials required to meet the objective of providing safe and effective medications. Nor is the state willing or able to mobilize the resources that would be necessary to undertake these tasks. Therefore, a tacit political decision is made to relinquish some authority to the drug manufacturers, especially with respect to information that forms the basis on which regulatory decisions are made. In this model, termed "clientele pluralism," the state relinquishes some of its authority to private-sector actors, who, in turn, pursue objectives with which officials are in broad agreement.

Despite their different origins, their different operating models, and differences in the financial resources and number of personnel, the regulatory decisions that these different authorities make are often quite similar and historically have favored the interests of the pharmaceutical industry.

Abraham[4] documented the situation in the USA in the mid-1970s involving a group of FDA reviewers. These reviewers told the US Congress that when they recommended the approval of a drug, their analyses were hardly ever challenged, but when they rejected an application their judgments were sometimes unjusti- fiably overruled. Furthermore, they claimed, that when they pointed out that applications had inadequate data to support approval, they experienced harass- ment and were removed from reviewing the file. These claims were upheld by a Review Panel on New Drug Regulation, which found that although the FDA had not been "dominated" by the pharmaceutical industry there had been inappropri- ate contacts between the FDA and industry. The panel did not undertake an analysis of the scientific literature pertaining to the drugs in question and so was not able to make a finding of bias in the scientific aspects of the drug approval process but did conclude that "a non-adversarial philosophy vis-à-vis drug com- panies ... brought a kind of pressure to approve drugs on more adversarially inclined reviewers."[4]

In Canada, that influence can be seen by looking at regulatory decisions made in the 1960s and 1970s regarding the benzodiazepine class of drugs. These in- clude products such as diazepam (Valium®), triazolam (Halcion®), and lorazepam (Ativan®). Lexchin[5] examined this topic and showed that there is strong circum- stantial evidence that these drugs were approved on the basis of inadequate clinical trials, resulting in them being indicated for conditions for which they were not useful, and that significant safety issues were ignored. These deficiencies in the regulatory process were magnified in the advertising of these products to phys- icians, thus contributing to inappropriate prescribing.

The 1968 Medicines Act established the Medicines Commission in the UK, but the Act itself foretold the type of relationship that was envisioned between government and industry. The health minister at the time assured critics of the new law that there was no need for clauses to safeguard industrial innovation because some of the members of the commission would be drawn from the industry. The first Chair of the Medicines Commission outlined his vision of the regulatory philosophy that should exist: one that would find a happy medium between the conflicting objec- tives of maintaining the well-being of the industry and the interests of public safety.[4] Medawar and Hardon[6] illustrate how that philosophy was applied in the case of the selective serotonin reuptake inhibitor (SSRI) group of antidepressants, in particular paroxetine (Seroxat®; in North America the trade name is Paxil®). The Medicines Commission and its successors consistently refused to accept mounting evidence that this group of drugs had frequent and serious side effects, and was associated with significant symptoms when patients tried to withdraw from their use.

User fees and deregulation

The FDA

Since the early 1990s, the relationship between the pharmaceutical industry and all regulatory agencies has, if anything, intensified, driven by user fees from industry and an atmosphere of deregulation.

In 1992, in response to industry complaints about slow approval times, the US Congress passed the Prescription Drug User Fee Act (PDUFA). Under the PDUFA companies began paying user fees to the FDA. However, these fees were specifically earmarked to hire new reviewers to speed up the approval of applications. The fees were contingent on the FDA meeting specific goals on timelines, and until the reauthorization of the PDUFA in 2002 none of the funds could be used to fund any other FDA activities, including those involving safety issues. User fees from companies now account for more than half of the money that is available to the agency for reviewing new drug applications.[7] As in Canada, there were dramatic effects from the injection of industry money. From 1993 to 2003 approval times for priority review drugs (drugs judged to have a significant therapeutic advantage over existing medications) dropped from 14.9 months to 6.7 months, while times for standard reviews declined from 27.2 months to 23.1 months.[7]

Besides speeding up drug approvals, the PDUFA seems to have changed the atmosphere within the FDA, with some people believing that reviewers' ability to conduct an impartial scientific assessment has been seriously impaired. The Washington-based Public Citizen's Health Research Group (HRG) surveyed FDA reviewers in 1998 for their reaction to the changes in the agency. Nineteen out of 53 medical officers identified a total of 27 new drugs in the previous three years that they thought should not have been approved but were; and 17 said that standards were "lower" or "much lower" than they had been three years previously.[8] A subsequent survey by the Office of Inspector General confirmed some of these findings. Although 64% of FDA respondents had confidence in FDA decisions regarding the safety of a drug, at the same time 40% who had been at the FDA for at least five years indicated that the review process had worsened during their tenure in terms of allowing for in-depth, science-based reviews. Moreover, 58% felt that the six months allocated for a priority review was inadequate, while 21% indicated that the work environment allowed for the expression of differing scientific opinions to little or no extent.[9]

Adding to these problems, the share of FDA funding and the resources available for activities other than drug approvals have substantially decreased: the proportion of the budget spent in these areas has fallen from 83% in 1992 to 71% in 2000. Mirroring this decline there has also been a decrease in the number of employees (full-time equivalents) from 7736 to 6571.[10] One former FDA reviewer is quoted as saying: "When I joined [the FDA], there was an absolute emphasis on safety. It is very, very clear that the emphasis now is getting drugs approved. To justify not getting them approved is considerably more difficult."[7]

The current culture in the FDA can be gauged by examining how the agency dealt with three different drugs and drug classes: troglitazone (Rezulin®), an oral drug for diabetes; the use of SSRI antidepressants in children; and rofecoxib (Vioxx®). The story of troglitazone has been told in a series of articles in the *Los Angeles Times*.[11] It was fast-tracked for approval by the FDA in the second half of 1996 despite the lack of concrete evidence that it would either help prevent the complications of diabetes or the death rate associated with the disease. In fact, the initial FDA reviewer of the product, Dr John Gueriguian, recognized that the drug offered little significant therapeutic advantage over existing therapies and recommended that it not be approved. Warner-Lambert, the makers of the drug, complained to Gueriguian's superior, Dr Murray Lumpkin, who removed Gueriguian from the file. The FDA also withheld Gueriguian's report about troglitazone from the advisory committee that considered whether or not to approve the drug, but did provide the report to executives of Warner-Lambert in advance of the committee meeting.[12]

Within nine months of being on the market it became apparent that troglitazone was causing liver failure and death in a number of users. For this reason the drug was withdrawn from the British market in December 1997, but it remained available in the USA for an additional 19 months. During that time the FDA, in association with Warner-Lambert, argued that the drug was essentially safe and that all that was required was additional liver monitoring to detect potential problems. This recommendation was being made without any evidence that this monitoring would be effective, or even that doctors would follow the recommendation. In fact, a subsequent study showed that fewer than 5% of patients received the recommended monitoring.[13]

The day the withdrawal was announced Lumpkin was still arguing for more safety warnings and against a ban. By that time, the drug was associated with 63 deaths from liver failure.

Researchers have estimated that between 2% and 6% of children and adolescents may suffer from depression.[14] Because of the relative lack of child psychiatrists many of these people are treated by general practitioners (GPs), who usually lack training in nondrug forms of therapy. Moreover, the large amount of promotion for psychotropic drugs means that it is this form of treatment that GPs usually reach for. Therefore, although the SSRI antidepressants had never been approved by either the TPD or the FDA for the treatment of depression in children or adolescents, during the 1990s and early 2000s doctors were increasingly turning to these drugs when faced with childhood depression. Indeed, there were a small number of published studies that indicated that these drugs could be beneficial. However, there was a larger group of unpublished studies that found that not only were these medications ineffectual but that they could also promote suicidal ideation in children and adolescents.[14]

Although these studies were unpublished, they had been made available to the FDA by the drug companies that sponsored them. The British regulatory authority, the Marketed Healthcare Products Regulatory Agency (MHRA; the successor to the Medicines Commission), also had access to these data and in August 2003 issued a strong warning to doctors not to prescribe these medications to children. (Although in both this case and that of Rezulin the British regulatory agency took action well before the FDA did, this should not imply that there are not serious problems in the way that drugs are regulated in the UK.) In early 2004, an FDA employee, Dr Andrew Mosholder, had reached the same conclusion as the MHRA and prepared a report recommending that the FDA take similar regulatory action. However, senior officials in the FDA prevented Mosholder from presenting his findings to a public FDA hearing on childhood depression that was considering what to do about this class of drugs.[15,16] The rationale offered by the FDA for its actions was that the meeting's purpose was only to set up the guidelines for analyzing the data. Moreover, FDA officials claimed that they were concerned that if Mosholder testified it "would be potentially harmful to public health as it might lead patients who were actually benefiting from the use of these drugs to quit taking them."[16] Instead, another FDA employee presented Mosholder's data but it took a second meeting eight months later and public testimony before the FDA finally took any action to restrict prescribing of these drugs to children.

The final drug to be considered is Vioxx. In many ways the events connected with this drug closely resemble what happened with the other two. The goal behind the development of this entire class of drugs was that they would suppress inflammation but without causing serious stomach problems, such as major bleeding or perforation. These side effects were seen in a small percentage of users of traditional nonsteroidal anti-inflammatory drugs (NSAIDs). The pivotal study on Vioxx confirmed that it did offer gastrointestinal protection compared to naproxen, one of the traditional NSAIDs. However, the rate of heart attacks in those taking Vioxx was five times that of those on naproxen despite the fact that people with recent cardiovascular events were excluded from the study.[17] This finding could only be regarded as tentative since the trial was not designed to look for untoward cardiovascular endpoints. Even though the FDA had these data in 1999, it took until February 2001 for the FDA Arthritis Advisory Committee to meet and discuss the potential cardiovascular risks associated with Vioxx. The reasons for this two-year delay are obscure.[18] In April 2002 the FDA did instruct Merck to include certain precautions about cardiovascular risks in its package insert, but did not try to negotiate with Merck to conduct a trial to establish the cardiovascular safety of Vioxx. This lapse in FDA behavior is especially troubling since by the summer of 2001 an epidemiological study had concluded that it was "mandatory to conduct a trial specifically assessing cardiovascular risk and benefit."[19] In the meantime, Merck was spending up to $135 million per year on direct-to-consumer advertising of Vioxx,[20] something that the FDA did little or nothing to interfere with. It was not until the fall of 2004 that Merck finally removed Vioxx from the market following confirmation of cardiovascular toxicity in a trial looking at the use of the drug for the prevention of bowel cancer.[21] Through the entire affair the attitude of the FDA seemed to be to wait passively for the bodies to accumulate.

The withdrawal of Vioxx was not the end of the involvement of the FDA with the drug. In the summer of 2004, before the meeting that lead to the withdrawal of Vioxx, Dr David Graham, a FDA epidemiologist, was analyzing the data about the drug. When he told his supervisors that his conclusion was that the drug was dangerous and should be removed from the market, they pressured him to change his conclusion because it was inconsistent with the official position of the FDA. In order to obtain permission to present his findings at an international conference, Graham said: "I changed them to a fair degree, and it caused me a great deal of mental anguish ... I did it because I thought if I didn't, there was no way that the data would see the light of day."[7] When Graham told his story to a US Senate committee investigating this affair, senior FDA officials dismissed his charges that the FDA failed to protect the public claiming that his assertions were "irresponsible."[22]

The TPD

Canada instituted user fees to help fund the TPD. Pharmaceutical companies are charged a fee for every application that they submit to market a new product. In addition, they pay an annual amount for each drug they have on the market. By 2000, half the cost of running the TPD was coming from industry.[23] In 1994, before money was coming from industry, it was taking on average 38 months to approve a new drug and about 50% of applications were receiving a positive decision. Within one year of industry money starting to come into the TPD, approval times were cut in half and by the late 1990s between 60% and 70% of applications were being approved.*

Approval times have become a high priority for the TPD to the extent that out of $40 million allocated in fiscal 2003–2004 to improve the regulatory system, $31.5 million went primarily to this goal.[24] However, only 9% of the new active substances (products never marketed before in any form) marketed in Canada qualify as either breakthrough products or significant therapeutic improvements.[25] The loudest and most influential voice calling for faster drug approvals comes from the brand-name industry. In a recently released document, Rx&D, the association representing nearly all of the multinational pharmaceutical companies operating in Canada, emphasizes the excessive length of time that it takes to get a drug approved.[26] From the point of view of returns on investment, the industry's preoccupation with timeliness makes perfect sense, but whether that applies when a public health point of view is adopted is questionable.

The apparent reorientation of the TPD in favor of business interests is further reflected in its Business Transformation Strategy (BTS) that is being implemented. The BTS was introduced in early 2003 and ''builds on the commitments made by the Government of Canada to 'speed up the regulatory process for drug approvals,' to move forward with a smart regulations strategy to accelerate reforms in key areas to promote health and sustainability, to contribute to innovation and economic growth, and to reduce the administrative burden on business.''[27]

One of the key phrases in the BTS is ''smart regulation.'' This means that Canada should ''regulate in a way that enhances the climate for investment and trust in the markets.''[28] While health is not ignored, the emphasis is clearly on creating a business-friendly environment. The shift from the precautionary principle to risk management is subtle but unmistakable. Realigning regulation to conform to the principles of smart regulation would not totally abandon the concept of precaution but it seems to imply that there would have to be a threat of serious or irreversible damage before it would come into play.

The Australian Therapeutic Goods Administration (TGA)

The Therapeutic Goods Administration (TGA) in Australia performs much the same function as does the FDA and the TPD in evaluating the evidence for new drugs and deciding on whether or not to allow new products on to the market. Lofgren and de Boer[29] have analyzed recent developments in the regulation and governance of pharmaceuticals in the Australian market.

---

*Information from annual TPD reports is available at www.hc-sc.gc.ca/hpfb-dgpsa/tpd-dpt/index_drugs_reports_annual_e.html#2003

Prior to the late 1980s, the Department of Health, through the TGA, was the main government department responsible for pharmaceutical policy. The TGA's position was to protect consumer welfare without primary concern for the profits of multinational drug manufacturers. However, this position started to be undermined with the establishment of a subsidy system operated by the Department of Industry aimed at encouraging investments in manufacturing, research and development, and exports. This new policy, with its more market-oriented view, was reinforced with the adoption of recommendations from the Baume Report, many of which were aimed at reducing review times. Cost recovery was introduced with the goal that 50% of the funding of the TGA should come from industry by 1996–1997, and full cost recovery began in 1998. Further alignment of the TGA with industry came with the report from the Industry Commission. According to Lofgren and de Boer:[29] "Its terms of reference signaled the reduction of processing times, that business should be relieved of unduly complicated regulatory requirements, and that more extensive use should be made of evaluation reports and decisions from overseas agencies."

Just as the FDA's actions and inaction concerning Vioxx served to highlight its conflicting relationship with industry, Vioxx also illustrates how the TGA is reluctant to intervene when there are serious potential safety issues around drugs. An epidemiological survey concluded that: "It is mandatory to conduct a trial specifically assessing cardiovascular risk and benefits of these agents [COX-2 inhibitors],"[19] but it then took the TGA 18 months before the Australian product information about Vioxx was altered. Even then the statement minimized the potential for harm from the drug (Agnes Vitry, personal communication, May 2005).

Some common threads

The recent history of all three of these agencies, especially how they were affected by the introduction of cost recovery or user fees, is consistent with principal–agent and capture theories which Lawson,[30] in a piece critical of the pharmaceutical industry and its ties to the FDA, cites in his analysis of the impact of user fees on the FDA. Principal–agent theory proposes that there is a relationship between a principal who has a task that needs to be performed and an agent who is contracted to do the task in exchange for compensation. Before the introduction of user fees, the principal was the public in all three countries and the agent was the relevant regulatory authority. However, since 1994 a new principal has been added: the pharmaceutical industry that is now providing a substantial fraction of the money needed to run the drug regulatory system. Regulatory capture theory asserts that over time regulators tend to become advocates for the industry they are supposed to regulate as a result of conflict avoidance and influence from the industry. The theory predicts that over time regulatory authorities will become less receptive to the needs of the public and will more closely align their missions with that of the pharmaceutical industry.[30]

The FDA approach to troglitazone, the SSRIs, and Vioxx, the TPD's embrace of smart regulation, and the TGA's weak response to Vioxx highlight how far these agencies have gone down the road to risk management as opposed to the precautionary approach, an agenda which is much more compatible with corporate interests than with public safety.

Postmarketing surveillance

In general, regulatory agencies give short shrift to postmarketing surveillance. The FDA, as one example, has a staff of about 100 people to analyze reports about possible adverse drug reaction reports[31] compared to 2300 employees who approve new drugs.[10] The conclusion in the previous paragraph is reinforced by looking at the attitude of the regulatory agencies towards postmarketing surveillance. In Canada, out of $40 million in new money that went into the regulatory system, only $2.5 million was spent improving the monitoring of drugs already on the market.[24] In the UK, a parliamentary inquiry into the pharmaceutical industry heard criticisms about the relatively weak emphasis that the MHRA puts on postmarketing studies.[32]

In the USA and the UK the authority to approve drugs on to the market and to remove them is concentrated in a single body. Recently, the FDA announced the creation of a Drug Safety Oversight Board that will advise on the management of drug safety issues within the Center for Drug Evaluation and Research (CDER), the arm of the FDA that approves new medications. The new Board will not have the power to remove drugs from the market; that authority will still rest with the CDER.[31] Canada does have a separate organization that monitors drugs on the market, the Marketed Health Products Directorate (MHPD), but it cannot order drugs off the market and must defer to the TPD. The *Lancet*, one of the world's leading medical journals, editorialized that "creating a board with only advisory powers on an issue as important as drug safety is unacceptable."[31]

Industry is strongly in favor of the speedy approval of new drugs as this will extend the length of time that the drug is on the market and still protected from competition by its patent. But the majority of the evidence shows that the push over recent years to approve drugs at a faster rate is associated with more removals for safety reasons after drugs are on the market. However, there are some studies that do not support this conclusion.[7]

The US General Accounting Office conducted a study on postapproval risks for drugs that had been approved by the FDA between 1976 and 1985. Out of 198 drugs for which data were available, 102 posed serious postapproval risks. Among drugs approved in fewer than four years, those that had serious postapproval risks had generally been approved in a shorter time than those without such risks.[33] Abraham and Davis[34] compared drug withdrawals in the UK and the USA in the period 1971–1992 and reported a ratio of 2.7:1 (24:9 drugs). Their explanation for the lower number of withdrawals in the USA was that the longer period spent examining the data in that country allowed regulators there to detect serious safety problems before products were marketed. Estimates suggest that for every one month reduction in a drug's review time there is a 1% increase in expected reports of adverse drug reaction (ADR) hospitalizations and a 2% increase in expected reports of ADR deaths.[35] In Canada the number of drugs withdrawn from the market for safety reasons more than doubled in the decade after 1993 compared to the two previous decades.[36]

The reluctance to devote significant resources to safety issues extends to postmarketing surveillance in general. In the European Union (EU), certain classes of drugs are approved centrally (i.e. for all member countries) by the European Medicines Agency (EMEA). Under exceptional circumstances, even if it is impossible to provide comprehensive test results at the time, the EMEA will still approve drugs. Although we would expect that these approvals would be conditional and include a requirement for postmarketing randomized clinical trials to provide the needed data, such is not the case. That type of trial is infrequently done and as a result the conditional status has only been revoked in four of the 18 cases where it was granted.[37]

Both the UK and the EU require new drugs to undergo an automatic five-year renewal, but in both jurisdictions little is done to ensure a comprehensive review and a reanalysis of the products' benefit-to-harm ratio.[32,37] Between 1991 and 2000, companies in the USA made 2400 postmarketing commitments to the FDA for studies on pharmaceuticals and 301 for biologics, but by 2002 only 37% and 15%, respectively, of these commitments had been fulfilled.[38] Whether or not regulatory agencies should rely on companies to carry out adequate postmarketing studies is also questionable. A review of 31 industry-initiated studies found that 22 were uncontrolled, only five reached their projected sample size, and 11 had been abandoned because of slow recruitment.[39]

Trials conducted to get drugs approved use a highly selected group of patients – those with clear-cut evidence of the disease in question, who are not taking other products, and who do not have other conditions that might interfere with an analysis of the efficacy of the product being tested. Drugs are also tested for relatively short periods of time. Once drugs are approved, they will typically be used in a much wider group of people and often for much longer periods of time. How these different populations will be affected by new drugs is usually unknown and sometimes the consequences can be disastrous, as exemplified by Vioxx. In this light, postmarketing studies take on increasing importance and the appearance that no agency is aggressively pushing for them to be done is highly disconcerting.

Transparency and conflict of interest

The FDA releases information on drug safety and efficacy along with comments from FDA reviewers. Information on manufacturing processes and trade secrets is not released. These data are posted on the FDA website where they are publicly available. However, the FDA's transparency has its limits: no information is released about a drug whose application is denied. This creates several potential pitfalls. New drugs not approved might be chemically related to products already on the market and reasons for the rejection of the former might point to unrecognized safety issues with the latter drugs. Companies might resubmit applications for new drugs and in such cases it is necessary to know why the drugs were initially turned down in order to be able to see if the deficiencies have been corrected. Drugs are often used off-label for uses that were never approved by the regulatory authority. It may be that the companies have applied for use for the indication in question but been refused for either reasons of safety or effectiveness. Without knowing about the failed application doctors will continue to prescribe and patients will continue to take a product that may be either harmful or ineffective in that particular situation.

The FDA approval process is potentially compromised by conflicts of interest, a subject that was discussed in the previous chapter by Joy Fraser. About 30% of the new drug applications that the FDA considers go to advisory committees composed of outside experts. These experts publicly debate the merits and demerits of the new drug and make recommendations about approval to the FDA. There are reports that some of the experts who sit on these committees have conflicts of interest. The House of Representatives Government Reform Committee has investigated allegations that certain physicians with multiple ties to manufacturers of heart drugs have been retained on the Cardiovascular and Renal Drugs Committee for extended periods in defiance of FDA regulations.[40] An analysis by the newspaper *USA Today* found that more than half of the experts who served on FDA advisory committees from January 1998 to June 2000 declared potential financial conflicts with the drug or policy being discussed or voted on. The federal agency is forbidden from using experts with financial conflicts unless a waiver is granted, usually on the grounds that the experts' value outweighs the seriousness of the conflict. The FDA grants these waivers routinely.[41]

In February 2005 an advisory committee voted 18 to 14 in favor of Vioxx returning to the market. Of the 32 members on the committee 10 had consulted for either Merck or the makers of other COX-2 inhibitors in recent years. All 10 of these people voted in favor of allowing Vioxx back; had they not voted the tally would have been 14 to eight against Vioxx.[42]

Despite its clear deficiencies, the USA actually has more transparency in its approval system than is the case in other countries. In Canada, all safety and efficacy data that the companies submit to get a new drug on the market are treated as commercially confidential and will only be released with the consent of the company involved, even if an Access to Information request has been filed.

The level of secrecy in the TPD has been criticized a number of times, including in a 2000 report by the ad hoc Committee on the Drug Review Process of Health, Canada's own Science Advisory Board.[43] The TPD response has been to develop what it calls a Summary Basis of Decision (SBD) that will summarize the key data on newly approved drugs and be publicly available.[44] An analysis of the quality and volume of data to be included in these SBDs has shown that they will be inadequate to ensure safe and rational use of new medications.[45]

The EMEA produces European Public Assessment Reports (EPARs) after a drug has been approved. These are supposed to reflect the assessment file submitted by the manufacturer, its analysis by the EMEA scientific advisory body, and the reasons underlying that body's opinion.[46] An analysis of nine EPARs issued during 1996–1997 found a striking lack of standard presentation of information in these documents. For instance, the reporting of clinical trials was not always clear and none of the nine EPARs mentioned references to published trials.[47] A subsequent analysis that covered all EPARs published in 1999 and 2000 revealed that the EPARs were not harmonized, reliable, or correctly updated.[46]

Some progress has recently been made in transparency in the EMEA. Under new European legislation financial interests of the EMEA experts and members of the EMEA management board must be declared on an annual basis and at each meeting declarations must be made of "specific interests which could be considered prejudicial to their independence with respect to the items on the agenda. These declarations shall be made available to the public." Also, under the same legislation, if the EMEA rejects a product for marketing, it must make the reasons for doing so publicly available.[48]

Regulation of drug promotion

The final area to be considered in this examination of regulatory function is drug promotion. Drugs must be accompanied by accurate objective information so that they will be prescribed appropriately by doctors and used appropriately by patients. Although the approaches that regulatory agencies take with regard to promotion are different, the results in terms of the quality of promotion are very much the same.

Amendments passed in 1962 to the Food, Drug, and Cosmetic Act gave the FDA jurisdiction over prescription drug promotional campaigns and materials. The FDA has defined its authority to cover any material issued by or sponsored by a drug manufacturer that falls within the legal definitions of labeling or advertising.[49]

However, the FDA is beset with limitations that undermine its ability to effectively control promotion. As a federal agency the FDA is chronically underfunded,[50] with the consequence that in the past, although the "vast majority" of promotional material submitted to the FDA division of drug advertising and labeling was considered "false and/or misleading," the FDA was able to take action in only 5% of cases because of lack of resources.[51] These limitations were highlighted in a 1992 review of 109 journal advertisements. These were evaluated using criteria based on FDA guidelines. Overall, independent expert reviewers would not have recommended publication of 28% of the advertisements and would have required major revisions in 34% of them.[52]

Although the FDA does not review ads before they are disseminated, manufacturers are obligated under the Food, Drug, and Cosmetic Act to submit copies of all advertisements to the FDA at the same time as they are first used commercially. The Division of Drug Marketing, Advertising, and Communications (DDMAC), the arm of the FDA that regulates promotion, continues to be overwhelmed by the volume of material it has to deal with. In fiscal 2002, the DDMAC had 39 full-time-equivalent positions to review approximately 34 000 pieces of promotional material.[53]

The shortage of personnel is best illustrated by the case of direct-to-consumer advertising (DTCA). In 1997, the FDA loosened the regulations around broadcast DTCA by removing the requirement for companies to provide all of the safety information on screen with the advertisement. Instead, companies henceforth needed only to mention major side effects and contraindications in audio or visual form and state where consumers may obtain additional information. As a consequence the amount spent on DTCA rose from US$1.07 billion in 1997 to US$3.24 billion in 2003.[53] But as of June 2002 the DDMAC had only five staff dedicated to reviewing DTCA material which included 248 television advertisements and an unknown but certainly large number of print advertisements.[54]

Along with inadequate resources to review DTCA, there was also a marked change in the willingness of the FDA to confront companies guilty of violations. When the FDA identifies a direct-to-consumer advertisement that is noncompliant with its regulations, it sends a letter asking that the company cease disseminating the advertisement. In the late 1990s the FDA was sending out between 100 and 150 such letters a year, but that number started to decline dramatically in 2000 so that by 2003 only 25 letters were sent.[55] Moreover, there was an increasing delay in sending out those few letters that were issued. Before 2002, regulatory letters were typically issued within one month of the FDA receiving the advertisements but by

2003 the average delay was 177 days.[56] The cause of the drop in enforcement actions and the lengthening delay appears to have been a November 2001 change in agency policy that required the FDA Chief Counsel to approve enforcement actions. At that time the Chief Counsel was Daniel Troy, who, prior to his appointment in August 2001, had represented the tobacco industry in its fight against FDA regulation and had opposed FDA efforts to restrict the promotion of drugs for unapproved uses.[7]

Most other countries have chosen to turn their regulatory authority over promotion to the pharmaceutical industry itself. As Lexchin and Kawachi[57] noted, there are two major drawbacks to government regulation: one financial, the other practical. Increasingly, fiscal pressures in almost all countries have prevented government agencies from effectively policing pharmaceutical promotion. Government regulatory agencies rarely have the resources to make it economically rational for individual firms *not* to cheat. The other major drawback to government regulation is a lack of necessary expertise compared to industry. Voluntary self-regulation therefore seems an attractive option because, lacking government–industry adversariness, it is a more flexible and cost-effective option. Government regulators also reason that in a highly competitive industry, the desire of individual companies to prevent competitors from gaining an edge can be harnessed to serve the public interest through a regime of voluntary self-regulation run by a trade association. However, although misleading advertising may to some degree inhibit competition, it is also far more often good for business.

New Zealand is the only other developed country that allows DTCA of prescription drugs. Industry practices are regulated by a Code of Therapeutic Advertising which is administered by the Advertising Standards Complaints Board (ASCB), a body appointed by the Advertising Standards Authority (ASA), an advertising industry body. Coney[58] gave an example of what happened when her organization, Women's Health Action Trust (WHAT), complained in 1999 about a direct-to-consumer advertisement. Although this complaint was ultimately upheld, it took six months for WHAT to be told that the complaint was successful. During this period WHAT was required to respond to several requests by the ASCB for more information, sign a waiver that it gave up any right "to take or continue any proceedings against the advertiser, publisher or broadcaster concerned," and adhere to a requirement not to make the result public before the ASA did. In addition to these onerous requirements on the part of complainants, Coney points out that the ASCB has limited powers. Its decisions are not binding or enforceable. The current executive director of the ASA says that it prefers voluntary compliance and an educational approach.

The Canadian government has chosen to turn over its regulatory authority to two bodies: the Pharmaceutical Advertising Advisory Board (PAAB), which controls print advertising, and the brand-name pharmaceutical industry (Rx&D), which regulates the behavior of its sales representatives and how company-sponsored continuing medical education is run. The codes for both the PAAB[59] and the Rx&D[60] operate under a reactive as opposed to a proactive style of regulation; that is, action is generally taken only upon receipt of complaints, rather than preventing breaches from occurring in the first place.

Neither code has effective sanctions where breaches have occurred. The PAAB has no authority to levy monetary sanctions, although it can require companies to pull offending advertisements, but by the time a complaint has been made and a ruling taken, the advertisement may be near to completing its run. The penalty for the third violation of the Rx&D code in a single year is a $15 000 fine; for large drug companies this is the equivalent of lunch money.

Neither code has a predefined period after which it needs to be reviewed; there was no major revision to the PAAB code between 1992 and 2004. The PAAB code does not have any specific provision about the type size for safety information, while detailed prescribing information does not have to be placed directly after the main body of the advertisement but can appear at the back of the journal. The Rx&D code does not require sales representatives to provide doctors with specific information about risks, contraindications, and warnings, and they do not have to leave a copy of the government-approved Official Product Monograph which provides detailed information about the drug.

Finally, self-regulation appears to be failing in the UK. There the Code of Practice of the Association of the British Pharmaceutical Industry (ABPI) is administered by the Prescription Medicines Code of Practice Authority (PMCPA), which receives funding from but operates independently of the APBI. The parliamentary committee investigating the pharmaceutical industry heard evidence that lead it to state: "The examples cited to us of breaches of advertising regulations, cover-up of negative medicines information and provision of misleading information to prescribers suggest that self-regulation is not working satisfactorily."[32]

Conclusion

The foregoing does not mean that regulatory authorities are totally aligned with the interests of the pharmaceutical industry. All agencies continue to make decisions that are of significant benefit to the general public. However, what should also be apparent is that when there is a choice to be made between public health and private profit, these agencies will typically favor private interests.

Favoring private interests means that resources that could be going into the healthcare system instead end up in the coffers of the pharmaceutical companies. When drugs are approved too quickly, safety problems may be missed; prescribing of drugs with major safety issues means more money being spent on doctor visits, testing, and hospitalizations for them. A lack of transparency in the approval process means that doctors do not have the necessary information to prescribe drugs properly and patients lack the knowledge about how to use them in the most appropriate way. Both situations contribute to wasteful expenditures for medicines. Misprescribing of both new and old drugs and the resulting consequences are furthered when little is done to investigate the risk–benefit profile of drugs once they are marketed. It is naïve to assume that once a drug has been initially approved that there is nothing further to be learned. Finally, the lack of control over the promotional excesses of the companies magnifies the problem as the message from the advertising is translated into enthusiastic use of unnecessary drugs. This is explored in the following chapter.

The problem with drug regulation is systemic; simply changing a few faces at the top level of the organization or tightening a few rules will not suffice to alter the modus operandi of these agencies.

The top priority must be to break the fiscal connection between the pharmaceutical industry and its regulators. There should be full and adequate public funding for the task of drug regulation. With the public paying the entire bill there cannot be any doubt about who the client of the agencies is. The experiment with deregulation should be ended. We need to recognize that drugs are unique products that must be treated differently than other consumer goods. If companies that make soap fail to self-regulate in an acceptable manner, the consequences are very different than if the same thing happens with pharmaceutical companies. The precautionary principle must be the prime force behind drug regulation, not risk management. Risk management is not acceptable when the consequences are dead patients.

In the case of countries other than the USA, there must be much greater transparency in the regulatory process so that it is evident how and why decisions are being made. The FDA needs to deal with the significant level of conflict of interest that exists with many of the outside experts that it uses on its expert advisory committees. All agencies have to be given the authority to mandate postmarketing surveillance studies and the resources to ensure that they are carried out. These additional resources can also be employed to strengthen their respective adverse drug reaction reporting systems. Control over drug promotion should be handed over to independent bodies that are established by legislatures, free of excessive industry influence, and that include health professionals and consumers. These bodies would establish and enforce regulations around promotion, pro-actively police promotion by monitoring a selection of all types, and have the power to impose penalties that are commensurate with violations. One concept that is useful here is a regulatory pyramid whereby initial violations are treated relatively leniently but subsequent ones incur increasingly harsh penalties that could include a ban on all promotion of the product for a period of time.

These proposals are only an initial outline of what needs to be done. Accomplishing these objectives will require generating political will.

References

1 Royal Society of Canada (2001) *Elements of Precaution: Recommendations for the Regulation of Food Biotechnology in Canada: An Expert Panel Report on the Future of Food Biotechnology.* Royal Society of Canada, Ottowa.
2 Wiktorowicz ME (2003) Emergent patterns in the regulation of pharmaceuticals: institutions and interests in the United States, Canada, Britain, and France. *J Health Polit Policy Law.* 28: 615–58.
3 Atkinson MM, Coleman WD (1989) *The State, Business, and Industrial Change in Canada.* University of Toronto Press, Toronto.
4 Abraham J (1995) *Science, Politics and the Pharmaceutical Industry: controversy and bias in drug regulation.* UCL Press, London.
5 Lexchin J (1998) The relationship between pharmaceutical regulation and inappropriate prescribing: the case of psychotropic drugs in Canada during the 1960s and early 1970s. *Int J Risk Safety Medicine.* 11: 49–59.
6 Medawar C, Hardon A (2004) *Medicines Out of Control? Antidepressants and the Conspiracy of Goodwill.* Aksant Academic Publishers, The Netherlands.
7 Okie S (2005) What ails the FDA? *N Engl J Med.* 352: 1063–6.
8 Lurie P, Wolfe SM (1998) *FDA Medical Officers Report Lower Standards Permit Dangerous Drug Approvals.* Public Citizen, Washington, DC.
9 Office of Inspector General (2003) *FDA's Review Process for New Drug Applications: a management review.* Department of Health and Human Services, Washington, DC.

10 General Accounting Office (2002) *Food and Drug Administration: effect of user fees on drug approval times, withdrawals, and other agency activities.* US General Accounting Office, Washington, DC.

11 Willman D (2002) The rise and fall of the killer drug Rezulin. *Los Angeles Times.* June 4.

12 Willman D (2002) FDA post-mortem finds drug approval problems. *Los Angeles Times.* November 16.

13 Graham DJ, Drinkard CR, Shatin D, Tsong Y, Burgess MJ (2001) Liver enzyme monitoring in patients treated with troglitazone. *JAMA.* **286**: 831–3.

14 Whittington C, Kendall T, Fonagy P, Cottrell D, Cotgrove A, Boddington E (2004) Selective serotonin reuptake inhibitors in childhood depression: systematic review of published versus unpublished data. *Lancet* **363**: 1341–5.

15 Diller L (2005) Fallout from the pharma scandals: the loss of doctors' credibility? *Hastings Cent Rep.* **35**: 28–9.

16 Koski G (2004) FDA and the life-sciences industry: business as usual? *Hastings Cent Rep.* **34**: 24–7.

17 Bombardier C, Laine L, Reicin A *et al.* (2000) Comparison of upper gastrointestinal toxicity of rofecoxib and naproxen in patients with rheumatoid arthritis. VIGOR study group. *N Engl Med.* **343**: 1520–8.

18 Topol EJ (2004) Failing the public health – rofecoxib, Merck, and the FFDA. *N Engl J Med. 351*: 1707–9.

19 Mukherjee DM, Nissen SE, Topol EJ (2001) Risk of cardiovascular events associated with selective COX-2 inhibitors. *JAMA.* **286**: 954–9.

20 Yuan Y, Duckwitz N (2002) Doctors & DTC. *Pharmaceutical Executive.* August: 1–7.

21 Merck & Co. (2004) Merck Announces Voluntary Worldwide Withdrawal of Vioxx® on September 30. Available from www.vioxx.com/rofecoxib/vioxx/consumer/index.jsp (accessed July 23, 2005).

22 Lenzer J (2004) FDA is incapable of protecting US 'against another Vioxx'. *BMJ.* **329**: 1253.

23 Health Canada (2001) *Departmental Performance 2000–2001.* November 8. Available from www.tbs-sct.gc.ca/rma/dpr/00–01/HCan00dpr/hcan0001dpr01_e.asp (accessed March 25, 2005).

24 Health Canada Public Policy Forum (2003) Improving Canada's Regulatory Process for Therapeutic Products: building the action plan: multi-stakeholder consultation. Available from www.ppforum.ca/ow/ow_e_05_2003/Presentation%20_Overview_of_Action_Plan (accessed July 6, 2004).

25 Patented Medicine Prices Review Board (2004) *Annual Report 2004.* Available from www.pmprb-cepmb.gc.ca/english/home.asp?x=1 (accessed August 5, 2005).

26 Rx&D (2002) *Improving Health through Innovation: a new deal for Canadians.* Rx&D, Ottawa.

27 Therapeutic Products Directorate (2004) *Business Transformation Progress Report.* Health Canada, Ottawa.

28 Government of Canada (2002) *The Canada We Want: speech from the throne to open the second session of the thirty-seventh parliament of Canada.* Available from www.pco-bcp.gc.ca/sft-ddt/docs/sft2002 (accessed February 15, 2004).

29 Lofgren H, de Boer R (2004) Pharmaceuticals in Australia: developments in regulation and governance. *Soc Sci Med.* **58**: 2397–407.

30 Lawson GW (2005) *Impact of User Fees (i.e. Drug Industry Fees) on Changes within the FDA.* College of Business and Public Management, University of La Verne. Available from www.fdastudy.com (accessed March 26, 2005).

31 Anon (2005) Safety concerns at the FDA. *Lancet.* **365**: 727–8.

32 House of Commons, Heath Committee (2005) *The Influence of the Pharmaceutical Industry: fourth report of session 2004–05, Vol 1.* The Stationery Office, London.

33 General Accounting Office (1990) *FDA Drug Review: postapproval risks 1976–85.* US General Accounting Office, Washington, DC.

34 Abraham J, Davis C (2002) *Mapping the Social and Political Dynamics of Drug Safety Withdrawals in the UK and the US. Final report to ESRC on Project R000237658.* Economic and Social Research Council, Brighton.

35 Olson MK (2002) Pharmaceutical policy change and the safety of new drugs. *J Law Economics.* **45**: 615–42.

36 Lexchin J (2005) Drug withdrawals from the Canadian market for safety reasons, 1963–2004. *Can Med Assoc J*. **172**: 765–7.

37 Garattini S, Bertele V (2001) Adjusting Europe's drug regulation to public health needs. *Lancet*. **358**: 64–7.

38 Food and Drug Administration (2002) *Report to Congress. Reports on Postmarketing Studies [FDAMA 30]*. Department of Health and Human Services, Washington, DC.

39 Waller PC, Wood SM, Langman MJS, Breckenridge AM, Rawlins MD (1992) Review of company post-marketing surveillance studies. *BMJ*. **304**: 1470–2.

40 Gribbin A (2001) House investigates panels involved with drug safety. *Washington Times*. June 18: A1.

41 Cauchon D (2000) Number of drug experts available is limited. Many waivers granted for those who have conflicts of interest. *USA Today*. September 25: A1.

42 Harris G, Berenson A (2005) 10 voters on panel backing pain pills had industry ties. *New York Times*. February 25.

43 Science Advisory Board Committee on the Drug Review Process (2000) *Report to Health Canada*. Available from www.hc-sc.gc.ca/sr-sr/alt_formats/ocs-besc/pdf/rep-rap/report_drp_e (accessed July 28, 2005).

44 Health Canada (2004) *Issues Analysis Summary: summary basis of decision – draft 7*. Health Canada, Ottawa. Available from www.hc-sc.gc.ca/dhp-mps/prodpharma/activit/ consultation/ias_dissemination_ra_diffusion_2_e.html (accessed November 23, 2004).

45 Lexchin J, Mintzes B (2004) Transparency in drug regulation: mirage or oasis? *Can Med Assoc J*. **171**: 1363–5.

46 Prescrire International (2002) *Reorienting European Medicines Policy*. Paris, June.

47 International Society of Drug Bulletins (1998) *ISBD Assessment of Nine European Public Assessment Reports Published by the European Medicines Evaluation Agency (EMEA)*. EMEA, Paris.

48 Prescrire International (2004) Medicines in Europe: the most important changes in the new legislation. *Prescrire International*. **158**: 1–158.

49 Kessler DA, Pines WL (1990) The federal regulation of prescription drug advertising and promotion. *JAMA*. **264**: 2409–15.

50 Slater EE (2005) Today's FDA. *N Engl J Med*. **352**: 293–7.

51 Anon (1989) FDA's drug promotion problems. *Scrip*. February 24: 14.

52 Wilkes MS, Doblin BH, Shapiro MF (1993) Pharmaceutical advertisements in leading medical journals: experts' assessments. *Ann Intern Med*. **116**: 912–9.

53 IMS Health (2003) *US Data Indices – Promotion, 2003*. Available from www.imshealth.com/ims/portal/front/indexC/0,2773,6599_44304752_0,00.html (accessed August 4, 2005).

54 General Accounting Office (2002) *FDA Oversight of Direct-to-Consumer Advertising has Limitations*. US General Accounting Office, Washington, DC.

55 Food and Drug Administration (2005) *Warning Letters and Notice of Violation Letters to Pharmaceutical Companies*. Department of Health and Human Services, January 12. Available from www.fda.gov/cder/warn (accessed August 4, 2005).

56 United States House of Representatives Committee on Government Reform – Minority Staff Special Investigations Division (2004) *FDA Enforcement Actions Against False and Misleading Prescription Drug Advertisements Declined in 2003: prepared for Rep. Henry A. Waxman*. Washington, DC.

57 Lexchin J, Kawachi I (1996) Voluntary codes of pharmaceutical marketing: controlling promotion or licensing deception. In: Davis P, ed. *Contested Ground: public purpose and private interest in the regulation of prescription drugs*. Oxford University Press, New York.

58 Coney S (2002) Direct-to-consumer advertising of prescription pharmaceuticals: a consumer perspective from New Zealand. *J Public Policy Marketing*. **21**: 213–23.

59 Pharmaceutical Advertising Advisory Board (2005) *Code of Advertising Acceptance*. PAAB, Pickering.

60 Canada's Research-Based Pharmaceutical Companies (2004) *Code of Marketing Practices*. Rx&D, Ottawa.

Chapter 5

The marketing of drugs: how drug companies manipulate the prescribing habits of doctors

Audrey Balay-Karperien, Norman J. Temple, and Joel Lexchin

Introduction

Global sales for the pharmaceutical industry are projected to reach about $645 billion in 2006.[1] As Big Pharma has continued to expand its unsurpassed global financial reign, increasing prescription drug spending has become a global concern. In Canada, drug spending has been growing rapidly in recent years: per capita spending (in constant 1997 Canadian dollars) increased 150% between 1985 and 2002.[2]

Increased spending is concentrated in only a few therapeutic categories, and these tend to be heavily marketed drugs.[3] Researchers and medical professionals have issued repeated warnings as to the excessive influence of drug companies in manipulating the prescribing habits of doctors, resulting in numerous research studies, articles, and books on the topic.[4-6] The essential argument is that drug companies, motivated by profit, are extremely successful in influencing doctors in ways that favor the pharmaceutical industry's financial interests over the public's health interests.

Chapter 7 examines the 10 most costly drugs prescribed in Canada. The estimates are that the drug bill for these products could be reduced by 55% simply by having doctors switch to lower-cost alternatives. This means that the Canadian public spends, directly or indirectly, almost a billion dollars a year in excess and unnecessary cash transfers to the pharmaceutical industry. And this figure will certainly be an order of magnitude larger in the USA. Supporting evidence for this came from another Canadian study.[7] Researchers investigated why spending on drugs in Canada doubled between 1996 and 2003. Their analysis showed that 80% of the increase was attributed to new, high-priced, patented, me-too drugs. This scandal of massive monetary waste is due, in no small part, to the marketing strategies described in this chapter. This makes one want to reach for mouthwash, eyewash, and antacid.

Interactions between doctors and the pharmaceutical industry

If doctors are going to treat people using the accumulated knowledge of science, they need to know about many things, including, of course, drugs. Doctors are also encouraged to learn to objectively assess new scientific data for themselves, but throughout their careers doctors also rely on the experience of trusted leaders and medical organizations to objectively distil the available and changing data into clinical guidelines. In reality, however, it is a system fraught with problems, mainly owing to the fact that practicing doctors are immersed in drug information provided to them by the pharmaceutical industry in a variety of ways.

Detailing

In hospitals and doctors' offices, sales representatives, known as "detailers," talk to doctors about the pharmaceutical industry's products and encourage doctors to prescribe them. Of \$22.1 billion spent by pharmaceutical companies on promotion and marketing to health professionals in 2003 in the USA, almost \$5.3 billion went to an army of sales representatives (reps).[8] From an industry perspective these people are a vital part of the marketing strategy. This is true around the world, although the tactics may vary from country to country, and even area to area within countries, depending on the strategies deemed most effective by the industry's impressive intelligence-gathering system.[9]

Drug reps can, for example, track and respond to changes in physician prescribing by purchasing information from the vast and detailed databases of prescription-tracking companies.[9] From the perspective of those on the receiving end detailing is both personalized and intense. The sales rep often assumes at once the roles of guest, generous friend, and proxy for a medical product company. Sales reps, for instance, sometimes in view of patients, engage doctors and their office staff in discussions that alternate between taking lunch orders and plugging the latest medical "breakthrough" offered by the drug company. In such a situation it is easy to lose sight of the fact that there is a fundamental conflict between the interests of doctors and those of the pharmaceutical industry (and of its sales reps).

In addition to being persuasive and pervasive, sales reps can be invasive. Marcia Angell,[4] a former editor-in-chief of the *New England Journal of Medicine*, described sales reps as "usually young, attractive, and extremely ingratiating." They are also numerous: Angell estimated that in 2001 there was one detailer employed by a drug company for every five or six practicing physicians in the USA, or about 100 000 in total. She also described how drug companies pay some doctors to allow sales reps to accompany them as they see patients, a rather disturbing practice that is clearly designed to build relationships that lead to business.

One reason many doctors give their time to sales reps is the expectation of useful information.[10,11] As noted above, sales reps have behind them a considerable amount of market research when they make visits, and they come prepared to deliver whatever sales pitch is most likely to achieve the object of the exercise. The efforts by sales reps to hawk drugs include providing reprints of articles, news of clinical trials, drug-specific educational material, and other distillations of information that appear to be helpful to a physician.[4-6,12]

Some insight into the tactics of sales reps can be gained from the website promoting the USA Pharma Sales Force Effectiveness Congress that took place in Philadelphia in May 2005.[13] The target audience was the supervisors of sales reps. Topics covered included the following.

- "Ways to increase physician receptivity to brand messages and the latest measures that can be taken to overcome third party formulary restrictions."
- "Detail effectiveness – assess how effective the quality of detail your reps deliver actually is and what can you do to make doctors more receptive to your products."
- "Top tips on overcoming the receptionists and ensuring your reps calls are valued as more than just a 'sample drop off.' "
- "Review how to ensure revenue winning skills are replicated across your whole sales force."

The cost of attending this two-day seminar was $1895.

Giving away free samples, known as "sampling," is a major activity of sales reps. Drug samples given out in the USA in 2003 had a retail value of $16.4 billion.[8] Granted, free drug samples can benefit some people without benefiting the drug industry if, for instance, they are used on a one-time basis for a problem that will not recur. Various researchers have confirmed that samples help some people by giving them access to appropriate therapy that they might not have been able to afford.[14,15] However, that is not the reason free samples are distributed, nor does it represent their primary effect. Rather, samples are available and can bring relatively immediate, apparently cost-free relief, pleasing patient and doctor, and the "brand loyalty" this creates, even if only for a short time, can lead patients or their insurers to increase spending. Taken with the enormous expenditures by the pharmaceutical industry on samples, these results highlight the fact that the point of free drugs is the same as that for free cheesecake samples at the local supermarket – they are not charity but enticements intended to increase demand for a specific product (potentially over a cheaper equivalent product).

These sales tactics are clearly focused on sales rather than health. This point is explicitly outlined in a course for doctors which is available on the American Medical Association's website.[16] One disparity the course points out is that whereas a physician's professional career comes with "an obligation to provide impartial medical care that will benefit patients or promote public health," a sales rep "engages in a for-profit commercial activity." The course illustrates that, by definition, a physician has "extensive scientific/medical training and expertise" and "uses knowledge for altruistic purposes," but an industry rep uses "product-specific, generally proprietary, knowledge for profit," is trained to provide "specific information about a product, often through promotion and advertising," and "may lack or be unable to disseminate relevant scientific knowledge due to restrictions (e.g. cannot discuss off-label applications)."

However much sales reps can be thought of as bringing information about new treatments to the attention of physicians, they can also act as bearers of logo-emblazoned coffee mugs, pens, textbooks, and tickets to sporting events, in addition to providing the free lunches noted above.[4,5] One of the problems with easily seen gifts, such as notepads, is that they may convey a message to patients that their physician approves a particular drug. Part of why free samples work may be simply a matter of proximity (the notepad is on the doctor's desk), but another likely reason is suggested by a body of socio-cultural research into reciprocity, which in this context means the tendency to give something in response to being given gifts.[17] According to John Abramson[5] the more lavish gifts offered to physicians by drug companies come with implicit strings attached, where failure to prescribe an overpriced drug might end the giving spree.

In a survey in the UK, for example, Watkins et al.[18] found that general practitioners (GPs) who have high prescribing costs were significantly more likely to see drug industry reps more frequently, prescribe new drugs more freely, and prescribe more readily to patients expecting a prescription. Another British study reported that sales reps are the most frequently used information source on drugs for GPs.[11] Studies have also indicated how different types of gift-giving by the pharmaceutical industry affect prescribing. In essence, the results of investigations into sampling show that, while variable, it can increase prescribing. To illustrate, Chew et al.[15] found that, in general, samples increase prescribing of sampled drugs. Similarly, in an online survey of 2300 physicians conducted by IMS Health, most (about 70%) of the respondents were "more likely to prescribe a brand-name medication in response to a patient request when they had a sample to give."[19] Likewise, Adair and Holmgren[14] reported that when resident physicians had access to drug samples, they were more likely to write prescriptions for heavily advertised drugs than for cheaper ones.

Not only is sampling designed to enhance sales but the evidence suggests that the availability of samples can have a negative effect on prescribing. When doctors in a family medicine center in the USA stopped accepting samples, their prescribing for hypertension improved dramatically.[20] In all likelihood this improvement was because the products being sampled were the newest (and most expensive) rather than the most appropriate.

Detailing is a good example of an industry practice that potentially fails public health. As noted, detailing can increase drug sales,[21] but the evidence suggests that the increase may not always translate into better treatment. Analyses of interactions between sales reps and doctors done in Australia, Finland, and France show that they rarely spontaneously mention safety information about their products, and frequently overemphasize their products' benefits.[22,23] A study in Germany found that only 6% of brochures given to doctors were scientifically supported by the literature.[24]

Probably as a result of the selective information that doctors receive, studies in various countries have consistently found that the more that they rely on information that they receive from detailers, the less appropriate is their prescribing.[25–28] This older work is supported by a recent report from the Netherlands where Muijrers et al.[29] concluded that "more frequent visits from pharmaceutical industry representatives was associated with a lower quality of prescribing."

Continuing medical education and symposia

Beneficence toward doctors on the part of pharmaceutical companies also comes in the form of "free education." This goes well beyond providing materials developed in order to promote a drug for a particular indication and into the realm of career enhancement by providing continuing medical education (CME). For doctors, CME is essential, not only as part of their remaining up to date, but also in many cases as a requirement for maintaining their licenses. Used properly it can, for example, warn about the dangers of antibiotic resistance caused by overprescribing, or educate physicians on the possible advantages of exercise and nutrition compared to many drugs. The problem occurs when learning is turned into sales spiels. Industry-sponsored CME, which poses an opportunity for the pharmaceutical industry to promote its products, can be well received by doctors as it saves them from having to pay for it.[30]

John Abramson,[5] a doctor who teaches primary care at Harvard Medical School, wrote that: "Drug companies understand precisely what it takes to persuade doctors to change their prescribing habits" and capitalize on that knowledge when preparing and making available accredited CME courses. One tactic he cites is akin to methods often associated with the marketing of such products as soft drinks and sportswear – drug companies sometimes endeavor to hire a key opinion leader who doctors see as trustworthy and use that person as endorser or presenter.

Turning CME into a marketing tool of the drug industry is the main complaint against industry-sponsored CME. This was highlighted in an editorial in the *Canadian Medical Association Journal*[31] that commented on some paid advertisements for CME that they were discontinuing; the editorial said:

> After receiving complaints from readers, we learned that the CME packages contravene guidelines established by the Canadian Medical Association and the US Accreditation Council for Continuing Medical Education. For example, the CME company and sponsor, not the course organizer, chooses the topics, design course content (which in some courses promotes use of the sponsor's drug) and selects the course leader, while financial conflicts of interest are not disclosed. In future, we will not include these CME inserts in our mailings of the print journal.

The effectiveness of CME as a means of promoting drugs was shown by investigators who reported increases in prescribing of a sponsoring company's product after doctors attended CME even though the company was not supposed to have any role in choosing the speakers at the event.[21,32] Even if the content of the CME is not biased in itself, the range of topics offered through company-supported CME is typically much more limited than CME offered by academic centers and is much more focused on drug therapy.[33]

A similar problem occurs when pharmaceutical companies are involved in medical symposia. Orlowski and Wateska[34] investigated the impact on prescribing when pharmaceutical firms gave all-expenses-paid trips to physicians so that they could attend symposia at which two new intravenous antibiotics for use in hospitalized patients were discussed. These researchers found that following the symposia there were significant increases in the prescribing patterns of both drugs investigated, as well as differences from national prescribing patterns. Perhaps the most telling finding of this study was that "the majority of physicians who attended the symposia believed that such enticements would not alter their prescribing patterns."

Drug advertising

Drug companies spent $448 million advertising their products in medical journals in the USA in 2003. Evidence indicates that the integrity of pharmaceutical advertisements directed at doctors is questionable. An analysis of 60 adverts that had appeared in the *British Medical Journal* between 1999 and 2001 demonstrated that drug advertising uses strong imagery to fabricate mythical associations between medical conditions and branded drugs, and that drug advertising manipulates readers' perceptions by subtle appeal to ancient and modern mythological foundations of humanism and Western psychology.[35] Cooper and Schriger[36] reviewed several hundred advertisements from the 1999 issues of 10 American medical journals. They determined that 58% of the original research cited in the pharmaceutical adverts was sponsored by or had an author affiliated with the product's manufacturer. By comparison, the figure was only 8% in a random selection of original research articles.

Direct-to-consumer advertising (DTCA) is a form of advertising of prescription drugs that is directed at the general public. Spending on DTCA in the USA reached $3.3 billion in 2003.[8] Several benefits of DTCA have been identified, for example encouraging patients to seek treatments for conditions that may otherwise go untreated. But there is a strong negative side. Several studies document that DTCA tends to increase prescribing. Murray and colleagues[37] reported the effects of DTCA on physicians and patients in the USA. They found that DTCA did produce some benefits but led people to request and sometimes receive prescriptions for the advertised drugs. In one study subjects were instructed to visit family physicians and general internists and pretend to have depression.[38] The investigators reported that the rate of prescribing of antidepressants was much higher when a specific brand was requested than when no brand was requested (a jump from 31% to 53% for "patients" with symptoms indicating major depression and from 10% to 55% for adjustment disorder). Murray et al.[39] carried out a survey of American physicians. Their findings indicate that 49% of requests by patients that are in response to DTCA are clinically inappropriate. Nevertheless, physicians filled 69% of requests they deemed clinically inappropriate. These findings are in line with those seen when consumers who had been exposed to direct-to-consumer adverts were questioned, as revealed in a study carried out by the Henry J Kaiser Family Foundation.[40] People were shown two televised drug advertisements. Although the subjects tended to feel the adverts are informative, at the same time they failed to retain some important information.

Mintzes, Lexchin, and colleagues[41] investigated DTCA and concluded: "... that more advertising leads to more requests for advertised medicines, and more prescriptions. If DTCA opens a conversation between patients and physicians, that conversation is highly likely to end with a prescription, often despite physician ambivalence about treatment choice."

Not surprisingly, physicians have a generally negative perception of DTCA. A survey of 760 American physicians voiced the opinion that such advertisements rarely provide enough information on cost (99% of respondents), alternative treatment options (95%), or adverse effects (55%).[42]

The marketing experts working for the pharmaceutical companies have clearly come to the conclusion that DTCA is effective at boosting sales. This is reflected in recent trends in how they spend their advertising budgets: whereas in 1997, in the USA, for every dollar spent on advertising in medical journals, the drug companies spent $2.10 on DTCA, by 2003 this had grown to $7.20.[8]

DTCA, it seems reasonable to conclude, increases prescribing, detracts from appropriate treatment, and undermines the doctor–patient relationship. In light of this, it is not surprising that DTCA is strongly opposed around the world with only

New Zealand and the USA allowing it. This appears to be a triumph of high-powered lobbying over sensible government.

Discussion

Doctors are continually bombarded, from multiple approaches, by sales-oriented tactics designed to change their prescribing habits. This is often based on information that is economical with the truth. And increasingly, at least in the USA and New Zealand, doctors are pressured by their patients who have been targeted with DTCA. This practice is especially inappropriate as patients are self-evidently not qualified to properly interpret this information.

The reason that the pharmaceutical industry puts such enormous resources into the marketing of drugs is, at risk of stating the obvious, to increase sales and thence profits. For instance, depending on brand size and launch date, for each additional dollar spent on detailing, the estimated return on investment ranges from $1.27 to $10.29; for journal advertising the range is $2.22 up to $6.86.[43]

Doctors are quick to claim that individually they are not affected by the volume of promotion directed their way, although they often express reservations about whether or not their colleagues may be susceptible.[44] However, despite these protestations the reality is that even doctors who say that they rely on objective scientific evidence in making their decisions about prescribing are often subconsciously biased by all of the promotional material that comes their way.[45,46]

Often, promotion is simply a case of a company trying to persuade doctors to prescribe their drug rather than the almost identical drug sold by a rival company. But we also find a great many cases of pharmaceutical companies attempting to shift prescribing patterns away from perfectly adequate, cheaper drugs of proven safety towards drugs that are far more expensive, may be newer (and therefore adverse side effects have yet to be identified), and which may be inappropriate for the patient. This is an important factor in the rapid cost inflation of medicine while doing little to improve public health.

One of these drugs is Crestor®, a member of a drug family known as statins. A doctor who decides to prescribe a statin has several to choose from. Some of these have been tested in long-term clinical trials and been shown to reduce the risk of heart disease. These are reviewed in Chapter 8. But Crestor is a "me-too drug;" it is a slight variation around the chemical structure of the other statins. While it has been shown in short-term trials to lower blood cholesterol, its effect on risk of heart disease has never been tested in a long-term clinical trial. This also means that we cannot say for sure how its safety profile compares with other statins. Despite this, and costing 50% more than generic statins, it has achieved tenth spot in Canada for all drugs, based on value of sales. The drug achieved this status thanks to heavy advertising, including frequent DTCA on American TV (which is often seen by viewers in Canada). The TV adverts do mention that the drug has not actually been shown to prevent heart disease, but the point is unlikely to be noticed by most members of the target audience. The *Lancet*, the British medical journal, ran an editorial in which it demanded that AstraZeneca, the manufacturer, should: "desist from this unprincipled campaign."[47]

A similar problem is seen with drugs for hypertension. These drugs are discussed in Chapter 7. The pharmaceutical companies have achieved considerable success in persuading doctors to prescribe calcium channel blockers and angiotensin-converting enzyme inhibitors: three of these drugs are among the top 10 most costly drugs prescribed in Canada. Yet, enormous cost reductions could be achieved by using diuretics, which, based on solid evidence, are just as effective and possibly safer.[48,49]

References

1 IMS Health (2005) Available from www.imshealth.com/ims/portal/front/articleC/ 0,2777,6599_3665_75719589,00.html (accessed November 11, 2005).
2 Canadian Institute for Health (2005) *Drug Expenditure in Canada: 1985–2004*. Canadian Institute for Health Information, Ottowa.
3 National Institute for Health Care Management Research and Educational Foundation (1999) *Factors Affecting the Growth of Prescription Drug Expenditures*. NIHCM, Washington, DC. Available from www.nihcm.org/FinalText3.PDF (accessed November 11, 2005).
4 Angell M (2004) *The Truth about the Drug Companies: how they deceive us and what to do about it*. Random House, New York.
5 Abramson J (2004) *Overdosed America: the broken promise of American medicine*. HarperCollins, New York.
6 Greider K (2003) *The Big Fix: how the pharmaceutical industry rips off American consumers*. Public Affairs, New York.
7 Morgan SG, Bassett KL, Wright JM *et al.* (2005) 'Breakthrough' drugs and growth in expenditure on prescription drugs in Canada. *BMJ*. 331: 815–6.
8 IMS Health (2004) www.imshealth.com/ims/portal/front/article. C/0,2777,6599_44304752_ 44889690,00.html (accessed November 11, 2005).
9 Skelton N, Haigh J, Wartenburg F and Hutton-Squire H (2005) A change of pitch. *European Pharmaceutical Executive*, March/April. Available from www.imshealth.com (accessed November 11, 2005).
10 McCormick BB, Tomlinson G, Brill-Edwards P and Detsky AS (2001) Effect of restricting contact between pharmaceutical company representatives and internal medicine residents on posttraining attitudes and behavior. *JAMA*. 286: 1994–9.
11 Prosser H and Walley T (2003) Understanding why GPs see pharmaceutical representatives: a qualitative interview study. *Br J Gen Pract*. 53: 305–11.
12 Klossner J and Newsom J (2005) Studying drug utilization by product indication. *Product Management Today*. 16: 16–17.
13 Eyeforpharma (2005) Available from www.eyeforpharma.com/salesusa05/program.shtml (accessed November 11, 2005).
14 Adair RF and Holmgren LR (2005) Do drug samples influence resident prescribing behavior? A randomized trial. *Am J Med*. 118: 881–4.
15 Chew LD, O'Young TS, Hazlet TK, Bradley KA, Maynard C and Lessler DS (2000) A physician survey of the effect of drug sample availability on physicians' behavior. *J Gen Intern Med*. 15: 478–83.
16 American Medical Association (2005) Medical vs Promotional Information. February. Available from www.ama-assn.org/ama/noindex/category/9696.html (accessed November 11, 2005).
17 Dana J and Loewenstein G (2003) A social science perspective on gifts to physicians from industry. *JAMA*. 290: 252–5.
18 Watkins C, Harvey I, Carthy P, Moore L, Robinson E and Brawn R (2003) Attitudes and behaviour of general practitioners and their prescribing costs: a national cross sectional survey. *Qual Saf Health Care*. 12: 29–34.
19 Yuan Y and Duckwitz N (2002) Doctors and DTC. *Pharmaceutical Executive*. 1: September. Available from http://mediwire.skyscape.com/main/Default.aspx?P=Content&ArticleID= 29973 (accessed November 11, 2005).
20 Boltri JM, Gordon ER and Vogel RL (2002) Effect of antihypertensive samples on physician prescribing patterns. *Fam Med*. 34: 729–31.
21 Wazana A (2000) Physicians and the pharmaceutical industry. Is a gift ever just a gift? *JAMA*. 283: 373–80.

22 Lexchin J (1997) What information do physicians receive from pharmaceutical representatives? *Can Fam Physician*. **43**: 941–5.

23 Anon (1999) Sales representatives: a damning report by Prescrire reps monitoring network. *Prescrire Int*. **8**: 86–9.

24 Kaiser K, Ewers H, Waltering A, Beckwermert D, Jennen C and Sawicki CT (2004) *Arznei Telegramm* **35**: 21–3. Available from www.di-em.de/data/at_2004_35_21.pdf (cited in: Tufts A (2004) Only 6% of drug advertising material is supported by evidence. *BMJ*. **328**: 485).

25 Berings D, Blondeel L and Habraken H (1994) The effect of industry-independent drug information on the prescribing of benzodiazepines in general practice. *Eur J Clin Pharm*. **46**: 501–5.

26 Bower AD and Burkett GL (1987) Family physicians and generic drugs: a study of recognition, information sources, prescribing attitudes, and practices. *J Fam Pract*. **24**: 612–6.

27 Powers RL, Halbritter KA, Arbogast JG, Neely JL and Williams AJ (1998) Do interactions with pharmaceutical representatives influence antihypertensive medication prescribing practices of family medicine and general internal medicine physicians. *J Gen Intern Med*. **13**(Supplement): 13.

28 Caudill TS, Johnson MS, Rich EC and McKinney WP (1996) Physicians, pharmaceutical sales representatives, and the cost of prescribing. *Arch Fam Med*. **5**: 201–6.

29 Muijrers PEM, Grol RP, Sijbrandij J, Janknegt R and Knottnerus JA (2005) Differences in prescribing between GPs. Impact of the cooperation with pharmacists and impact of visits from pharmaceutical industry representatives. *Fam Pract*. **22**: 624–30.

30 Marlow B (2004) The future sponsorship of CME in Canada: industry, government, physicians or a blend? *Can Med Assoc J*. **171**: 150–1.

31 Anon (2004) What's wrong with CME? *Can Med Assoc J*. **170**: 917.

32 Bowman MA and Pearle DL (1988) Changes in drug prescribing patterns related to commercial company funding of continuing medical education. *J Contin Educ Health Prof*. **8**: 13–20.

33 Katz HP, Goldfinger SE and Fletcher SW (2002) Academia-industry collaboration in continuing medical education: description of two approaches. *J Contin Educ Health Prof*. **22**: 43–54.

34 Orlowski JP and Wateska L (1992) The effects of pharmaceutical firm enticements on physician prescribing patterns. There's no such thing as a free lunch. *Chest*. **102**: 270–3.

35 Scott T, Stanford N and Thompson DR (2004) Killing me softly: myth in pharmaceutical advertising. *BMJ*. **329**: 1484–7.

36 Cooper RJ and Schriger DL (2005) The availability of references and the sponsorship of original research cited in pharmaceutical advertisements. *Can Med Assoc J*. **172**: 487–91.

37 Murray E, Lo B, Pollack L, Donelan K and Lee K (2004) Direct-to-consumer advertising: public perceptions of its effects on health behaviors, health care, and the doctor–patient relationship. *J Am Board Fam Pract*. **17**: 6–18.

38 Kravitz RL, Epstein RM, Feldman MD *et al*. (2005) Influence of patients' requests for direct-to-consumer advertised antidepressants: a randomized controlled trial. *JAMA*. **293**: 1995–2002.

39 Murray E, Lo B, Pollack L, Donelan K and Lee K (2003) Direct-to-consumer advertising: physicians' views of its effects on quality of care and the doctor–patient relationship. *J Am Board Fam Pract*. **16**: 513–24.

40 Kaiser Family Foundation (2001) *Understanding the Effects of Direct-to-Consumer Prescription Drug Advertising*. Kaiser Family Foundation, Kenlo Park, CA.

41 Mintzes B, Barer ML, Kravitz RL *et al*. (2003) How does direct-to-consumer advertising (DTCA) affect prescribing? A survey in primary care environments with and without legal DTCA. *Can Med Assoc J*. **169**: 405–12.

42 Robinson AR, Hohmann KB, Rifkin JI *et al*. (2004) Direct-to-consumer pharmaceutical advertising: physician and public opinion and potential effects on the physician–patient relationship. *Arch Intern Med*. **164**: 427–32.

43 Neslin S (2001) ROI analysis of pharmaceutical promotion (RAPP): an independent study. Presented on May 22, 2001. Available from www.rxpromoroi.org/rapp/exec_sum.html (accessed November 20, 2005).

44 Steinman MA, Shlipak MG and McPhee SJ (2001) Of principles and pens: attitudes and practices of medicine house staff toward pharmaceutical industry promotions. *Am J Med*. **110**: 551–7.

45 Avorn J, Chen M and Hartley R (1982) Scientific versus commercial sources of influence on the prescribing behavior of physicians. *Am J Med.* **73**: 4–8.

46 Greenwood J (1989) *Pharmaceutical Representatives and the Prescribing of Drugs by Family Doctors.* PhD Thesis, Nottingham University, Nottingham.

47 Anon (2003) The statin wars: why AstraZeneca must retreat. *Lancet.* **362**: 1341.

48 The ALLHAT Officers and Coordinators for the ALLHAT Collaborative Research Group (2002) Major outcomes in high-risk hypertensive patients randomized to angiotensin-converting enzyme inhibitor or calcium channel blocker vs diuretic: the antihypertensive and lipid-lowering treatment to prevent heart attack trial (ALLHAT). *JAMA.* **288**: 2981–97.

49 Whelton PK, Barzilay J, Cushman WC *et al.* (2005) Clinical outcomes in antihypertensive treatment of type 2 diabetes, impaired fasting glucose concentration, and normoglycemia: Antihypertensive and Lipid-Lowering Treatment to Prevent Heart Attack Trial (ALLHAT). *Arch Intern Med.* **165**: 1401–9.

Chapter 6

Pricing pharmaceutical drugs in the USA

Donald W. Light

Introduction

Pricing drugs in the USA has become the object of widespread consumer objection, extensive federal and state efforts to lower prices, the introduction of wholesale management companies, and a massive addition of coverage for prescription drugs under Medicare but at high prices and substantial profits for all involved. To get an independent sense of how high American prices are one can look at the report by the Productivity Commission of Australia[1] that compared drug prices in eight countries. The Commission took pains to obtain comparable prices in each country and found that the lowest US prices were about double those in any of the other affluent countries. For "me-too" drugs, prices in the massive American market were almost three times those in little Australia. The USA also had far more patents on a given drug than did other countries, what have become known as "patent thickets" that impede innovation. The commission also found that prices varied much more in the USA, and in this chapter I explain why.

Pricing patented drugs is a highly secretive and sophisticated craft, practiced by the major firms together with specialist pricing companies hired by them. Yet framing these secretive practices are laws and regulations resulting from politics and state actions. Perhaps no other industry so depends on the welfare of the state for its high prices and profits. Only now and then is one allowed to see how state protections and incentives are used to charge far more than cost.

Low costs, huge mark-ups

One informative incident is the current epidemic of fear over the avian flu and the desperate rush to stockpile Tamiflu®, the only known drug that might weaken the impact of the flu, though mutated strains reduce that possibility. Roche holds the patent, and up to at least October 2005 was extremely reluctant to license rights for others to manufacture it, even though it admits it lacks the capacity to come close to the size of orders by governments.[2] Although no cases have been detected in the West and only hundreds in China, the avian flu is predicted to cause 20–47 million Americans to become sick, leading to 314 000–734 000 hospitalizations, and 89 000–207 000 deaths. Similar projections are creating a global policy panic. One proposal before the US Congress would buy 20 million doses for $1.2 billion. (Since treatment consists of two pills a day for five days, which two million people would get it?) This price of $60 a dose compares to the retail price at my local drugstore of $9.95 a pill. Perhaps Congress should buy their 20 million doses from drugstores and save 80% of taxpayers' money.

Meantime, a *New York Times* reporter found that "Roche pays $1.85 for each kilogram of shikimic acid," the active ingredient, and uses 1.3 grams in a capsule.[3] If you do the maths, that comes to a quarter of a cent per dose. The rest of the process might raise the cost to a dollar a dose. Given no need to do any marketing, Roche would then stand to recover its costs of $20 million and make a profit of $1.18 billion or 98% gross profit on the sale. Roche emphasizes that the manufacturing is complex; but the Chair of Cipla, a sophisticated Indian manufacturer that meets stringent quality standards and that played a legendary role in manufacturing complex drugs for AIDS at low cost, said: "I don't think the chemistry is such a big issue." Once again, Cipla plans to manufacture a generic version, and once again Cipla is likely to show the world that vital drugs can be sold at a fraction of Western prices while still making a good profit. Missing from this argument is the need to recover the very high costs of research and development (R&D), but these too are much lower than claimed, as explained below.

High prices for products that suffering or dying patients need has made the pricing of drugs very controversial. For example, when America faced the threat of anthrax after the terrorist attack on the World Trade Center, the new Secretary of Health, "Tommy" Thompson, decided to buy large stocks of Cipro®, the most effective antidote. Bayer held the patent on the drug and stretched the law by paying a generic manufacturer $25 million a year to delay a generic version from going on the US market, where it was the only company allowed to sell the drug.[4] Legal monopolies lead companies to do anything to extend them, even if the high prices make the medicine inaccessible to patients who need it.

Bayer said its average wholesale price was $4.67 a pill. Patients or frightened citizens who wanted to buy the drug would pay the retail price of $6.00 a pill. Then a reporter disclosed that Bayer sold Cipro to some US government programs for $1.83 – less than half the stated wholesale price.[5] For 100 million pills, Thompson thought that was too much. Bayer balked, and Thompson threatened to have Congress break its patent on grounds of a public health emergency. The irony of doing so, at the same time that the USA was taking a hard line toward insisting on patent protections worldwide did not escape notice. Bayer conceded to 95 cents a pill for an order of 100 million, a 40% reduction of its rock-bottom price for government purchasers that Thompson said had "shocked" the company.[6] It further agreed to 85 cents a pill on the second 100 million and 75 cents on the third 100 million. The agreement was treated as a triumph of hard bargaining for the American people and a graphic illustration of how the new administration could drive down prices and get value for taxpayers' money.

Then, the *Washington Post* obtained an internal document showing that Bayer was already selling Cipro to a federal program for hospitals and clinics treating the poor for 43 cents a pill, less than half what Tommy Thompson paid on the first 100 million.[7] This raised disturbing questions. If the Secretary of Health, as chief negotiator for the nation, did not know this was he misinformed, not well briefed, or lax in his diligence? Or did he know and paid more than double an existing government price, waste taxpayers' money, give Bayer a windfall profit, and present the results as a triumph of hard bargaining? Why did the government not buy the 300 million pills for 43 cents? Why were some contracts for $0.43, others for $1.83, and this one for 75–95 cents? This seems to reflect the ability of drug companies to segment markets, even within one large buyer.

The pricing game for Cipro, however, was not over, as seen in Figure 6.1. Before Thompson made his contract with Bayer Ranbaxy and two other generic manufacturers offered to sell Cipro in large volume for less than half of Bayer's "sacrifice" price.[5] Their own price for Cipro in India, with profits, was 30 cents.[5] The quality of Ranbaxy, Cipla, and some other Indian manufacturers is high and their manufacturing quality certified by the FDA as an overseas supplier. This reflects the mature pharmaceutical industry in India that has been developed over the past 30 years. The *Wall Street Journal* did not think Thompson had struck much of a bargain. With no marketing and little overhead on single sales of 100 million pills each, Bayer made a very profitable contract while appearing to be shocked by its "rock-bottom" concession to Tommy Thompson.[8] If Cipro costs 5 cents in volume to produce, then 95 cents is 19 times cost, the average wholesale price is 93 times cost, and the retail price of $6.00 a pill represents a mark-up of 12 000%. Mark-ups of 40–100 times costs appear to be common.

The same disparities between costs and prices have occurred in drugs for AIDS, such as AZT. As the lawsuit by the AIDS Healthcare Foundation against GlaxoSmithKline documents, the company had no research and development costs to recover because AZT was developed under grants supported by taxpayers through the NIH.[9] Yet the initial monopoly price was set at $10 000–$12 000 a year. Under intense public pressure, however, prices dropped sharply, and eventually the Clinton Foundation negotiated a price of $140. It appears that the actual cost of production is about $100 a year. Thus, the initial charge to desperate patients appears to be about 100 times manufacturing cost, and it still is for some patients in the USA.

Pricing drugs in what is described as the open, American free market results, paradoxically, in the highest prices in the world. The term "free market" seems to mean the ability to price free of a real market, because of government protection. The industry rails against government "price controls" in Canada and Europe, where a price board often negotiates volume discount prices with companies, but corporate price controls prevail in the USA. This is why drug companies are able, uniquely in America, to raise their world-high prices every year.[10-12] The industry, and professors of economics, always say the prices are set by "the market," but markets are politically constructed realities. With drugs the pharmaceutical industry constructs secret, segmented markets in which they control prices internally. Professors of economics would be more accurate if they said that prices for patented drugs are set in politically constructed markets, which in this case are usually structured to be monopolies or oligopolies where little price competition takes place.

To write an analysis of pricing drugs in America seems almost impossible, so much is shrouded in secrecy and segmented to minimize price competition. Current literature is not helpful. For example, the description of the US pricing system for a London School of Economics project is entirely devoted to government purchasing, because that is the only place where the author could find information.[13] The Congressional Research Service Report for Congress on factors influencing the pricing of drugs states: "The market power of large, research-based pharmaceutical manufacturers is offset by that of the generic drug producers and large payers for prescription drugs: the insurance companies, governments, and various health care providers … ."[14] This misrepresents the lopsided imbalance of market power evident in US prices being higher than the highest price set in other affluent

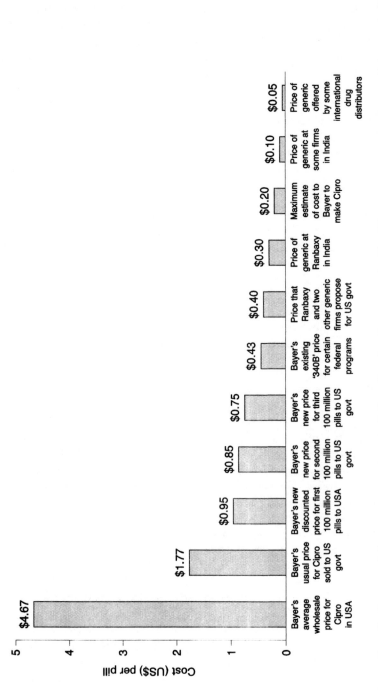

Figure 6.1 Even allegedly discounted drug prices promise windfall profits: the Cipro example. The US government recently gave Bayer a windfall profit of over $70 million by paying far more than the actual cost of making 100 million doses of the antibiotic Cipro®. (Sources: Harris G (2001) Bayer's Cipro will be profitable, even on discount deal with US. *Wall Street Journal*, October 26; Vedantam S (2001) HHS's varying costs for Cipro criticized. *Washington Post*, October 26. ©2002 Deborah Scholar and Alan Sagar, Boston University, School of Public Health, reproduced with permission. You are free to reprint this. Please credit the authors.)

countries: the lowest published US price set, the Federal Supply Schedule, is 69% higher than Canadian prices and double prices in Italy or France, for the same drugs.[15] In the "competitive" US market, generic use is also among the lowest, and overall costs have been increasing the most.

The pricing model of pharmaceutical companies

Most professional articles on pricing drugs focus on cataloging patterns or delving into the technicalities of pricing theory. Such articles can be useful.[16] Different rules may operate in countries like Canada where drug prices are lower and hardly rise at all (less than 0.5% per year since 1993). In the USA, drug companies have been raising their high, unmanaged prices on pre-existing drugs each year as well as getting physicians and patients to switch to new, more costly drugs and to expand use.[11,12,17] Thus pricing is one part of a comprehensive marketing strategy. We now turn to the actual kind of model used by companies to calculate prices.

How prices are decided

Companies and their experts hold that pricing is based on value and therefore all new drugs add value, otherwise they would not sell. The value of a new drug is made up of the *reference value*, the price of the best alternative, and the added or *differential value* of the new drug. There can also be negative differential value if a new drug with a more effective main effect might have more adverse side effects or a less convenient dosage regime.[18] The goal is to maximize the size of the differential value and the demand for it.

Since patients are the other end-user, along with physicians, one can appreciate the importance of direct-to-consumer marketing so as to reach patients as effectively as companies reach physicians through their legions of sales reps. What industry literature does not emphasize much is that "value" can be created and inflated. Or, rather, that need itself can be created. Take Viagra®, for example. Its promotion went from featuring Bob Dole as a senior citizen who would like to perform better, to men in their forties who wanted to perform as they did in their twenties. Is this a need? A desire? Is it enhancement, or a "cure" for a "disorder" that increases with age? Another kind of example is Vioxx®. Its only benefit over a generic costing about 100 times less was the reduction of adverse gastro-intestinal reactions that affect about 7% of the population. Its clinically appropriate sales should have been 7% of all sales of this type of drug. But by leading people to believe that it was superior in general and eliminated the chance of an unlikely adverse reaction, and by heavy marketing to physicians, Merck greatly expanded the perceived differential value and use of the drug.

Through these and other strategies corporate price experts develop a "value dossier" which justifies a higher price and greater use. Not included in this pricing model, but directly relevant to its key variables, are inducing larger market size, brand loyalty, differential value, patterns of repeat purchasing, inducements and persuasive charm with physicians, free samples, and low prices to hospitals to get patients started on a drug they will use after discharge. One distinct advantage in testing drugs against a placebo is that one can claim greater differential value than one could with testing against the best in a therapeutic class, and thus a high price through "indirect comparative analysis".[18] Another related strategy not mentioned is to recruit leading clinicians in the relevant specialty at academic and other leading centers to give paid talks in courses (almost always now funded by pharmaceutical firms) in which they indicate their preference for the drug being marketed. This leads to the concerns of NoFreeLunch, a website that addresses the corruption of independent clinical judgment and the commercialization of the medical profession.

The logic of the corporate pricing model is based on two convictions:

- all drugs enhance the quality or longevity of life
- the more drugs you take, the healthier you will be.

Part of pricing is defining what the product is, what indications it can be used for, where it is used in the overall treatment regime, which kinds of providers prescribe it and in what settings, and the mode of administration. To this I would add the factor of the patient, both as payer and source of increased demand, and the nature of the indications. Viagra, for example, is predominantly a lifestyle drug for which patient demand is critical to market size, that can be prescribed by any physician, and self-administered at home. Contrast this to Gleevec®, a very powerful drug that needs close monitoring and is usually prescribed by a subspecialist in hospitalized patients who are on their way to dying.

The heart of the pricing model is the calculation of net present value (NPV) over the full product development and marketing lifecycle of a product, as shown in Figure 6.2.

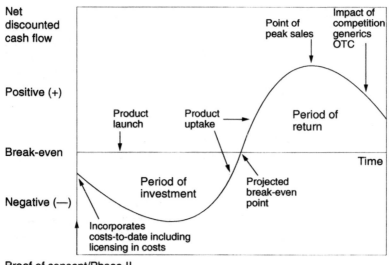

Figure 6.2 A hypothetical cashflow curve for a pharmaceutical product. A long initial period of negative cashflow is typical; a high gross margin is required to recoup and provide a return on this investment. OTC, over-the-counter.

According to a senior pricing authority "... a high gross margin is needed if the product's net present value (NPV) is to be positive. This is because there might be 10 or more years of research and development costs, without any revenue generation, before the product begins to generate gross margins." Notice on the left of this figure that costs start with Phase II trials and that all research and development costs from discovery through Phase I are quite modest. Then notice that most of the fixed costs occur after product launch. These are not R&D costs; rather, they are the huge marketing budget plus postlaunch Phase IV trials. The objective is to get doctors to write more prescriptions for the drug than they would just from its merits and from media reports. The curve in the figure reflects what corporate reports show, that the large pharmaceutical firms spend about three times more on marketing and handsomely rewarding administrators (with bonuses tied to stock price gains) than for R&D. Also, notice that the returns are equal to or less than the size of the investment: implying that the company took a huge gamble just to break even. If this were true, company executives would do better just investing the original money in a balanced portfolio and taking a lot of vacation time.

The myth of immense research costs

Key to pricing and the NPV model is the allegedly huge direct costs of R&D that have to be recovered. A chief consultant to Pfizer was Frederick "Mike" Shearer, a brilliant economist at Harvard, who became an eminent figure in the profession. He explained to me that he advised, whenever critics bring up prices, emphasize the cost of research.[19] This advice was the central rationale for 50 years, worth billions in sustaining high prices.

The need to recover ever-higher estimates of R&D costs has played a central role in every extension of the industry's ability to set prices in protected markets. The industry's lobbyists and their large public relations network write reports and "news" articles that are readily published as facts with no verifiable evidence. They have persuaded everyone that innovative drugs will not be possible unless companies are allowed to set high prices. Like rumors, if you keep repeating a claim, it assumes the status of a fact. In essence, the industry says over and over, "I can't show you our proprietary data, but believe me, R&D costs are astronomical." Pharmaceutical executives love to regale listeners with awe-inspiring tales of immense costs, just for one trial; yet based on even more routine industry data the tale is as long as an elephant's tail.

The unverifiable claim is that average cost for R&D per drug is currently around $1–$1.5 billion. This average figure, like most pharma-facts, come from hired academics, especially economists, who take secret, self-reported data from companies and then build econometric models to come up with large estimates. Even if true, there is no way to link this claim to sales or gross profits because detailed figures per drug are never revealed, and all three numbers vary by a factor of 10 across all drugs. An average of such wide variation is meaningless.

The basis of the current authoritative estimate (aside from those done by commercial consulting firms) uses confidential data submitted to one of the industry's principal policy research centers.[20] It was published in the *Journal of Health Economics* over a year after the results were released in a worldwide press conference organized by the industry. Light and Warburton[21] identified several basic flaws in this estimation, including: the sampling of the firms was not random and the sample was too small to be statistically reliable (10 firms); the nature of the firms was not revealed and there could be considerable variability among them; the cost figures were from another data set and related to the first set in questionable ways; the drugs chosen were by far the most costly subset of all drugs reviewed by the FDA; and the cost figures were subject to several kinds of variability. Although the paper was called "The Price of Innovation," the authors had no good data on the cost of actual innovation, that is, the cost of basic research to discover new drugs. The authors vigorously protested that these problems did not exist or that they had adequately addressed them.[22] In a full reanalysis of the world's most cited and influential article on the cost of innovation, Warburton and Light have found that on the basis of the industry's own data, the estimated average cost of R&D was one-tenth the estimate claimed by the industry.

Regardless how much R&D costs, the key question is how long does it take for companies to earn it back? In 2005, Joel Lexchin and I published a closely documented article showing that pharmaceutical companies earn back all R&D costs each year, in Canada and Europe, with good profits, just from sales in those countries.[23] Companies charge super-prices in the USA for super profits just because they can get away with it. The evidence comes from the industry's own data in easily accessible reports. Thus it appears that companies have been misrepresenting their own data for decades. The claim that US prices are high because foreign prices do not even cover R&D costs is not supported. This "free-rider" claim is also based on the erroneous claim that each country is responsible for prices that recover companies' R&D country in that country. In fact almost all new drugs are marketed worldwide, so it makes little difference where a drug is discovered.

Our article also used data from the National Science Foundation to calculate that large pharmaceutical firms devote 1.3% net of domestic income from sales to basic research. Thus the slogan "Today's Medicines Pay for Tomorrow's Miracles" is only true at a rate of 1.3 cents per dollar.

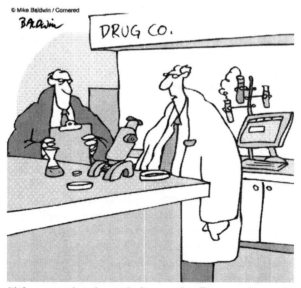

"It's a major breakthrough. But we're still years away from being able to justify the outrageous cost per pill."

Other aspects of pricing

Pricing is significantly influenced by patents and other forms of protection from price competition. While the NPV model justifies high prices despite a long period of protection, I have indicated the ways in which the key variables and multipliers are open to exaggeration and are unrealistically high in the cases where independent analyses can be made.

Patents are intended to serve as a temporary stay from price competition to reward innovators, but also to make them realize that they must innovate again if they want another patent. Goozner's[24] detailed accounts are sobering: of how the long protection that patents provide has led innovative young companies to become more like legal patent protection firms that happen to do some research, obsessed with how to extend their monopoly protection. Many cases and lawsuits document the diverse techniques for extending patents and other protections from price competition, all of which extend the lifecycle of the initial new drug by many years. This is another important error in Figure 6.2 and in all articles on the lifecycles of drugs and the profits of pharmaceutical companies. These lifecycle curves are based on just the sales curve of the initial patent without extensions of market protection by adding subsequent patents, patenting variations on the original molecule, invoking data exclusivity, or gaining two and a half years more protection just by filing a lawsuit, even if devoid of merit, against a generic company that has applied to compete. If the price of a new drug was based on the full lifecycle, all costs would be recovered and a reasonable profit earned while charging much lower prices.

As a commercially constructed reality, prices are numeric manifestations of values, goals, and strategies. The econometrics of pricing gives its deeper nature a pseudo-scientific gloss, a pretence that for $600 an hour each, a team of PhDs can come up with the "right price." Pricing is surrounded by ideology and mystique, by business fashions, by power plays, and by avarice, the extraction of maximum profit from this social good. Pricing, in short, is a drama of rivalry, stealth, triumph, and tragedy. The use of double-speak advances the cause by leading the listener or reader to think the opposite of what is meant. Figure 6.3 lists some key examples.

"Free market pricing"	=	Pricing free of market competition
Regulations	=	Those anti-free enterprise things on which drug companies entirely depend
"Reference pricing"		Pricing low for low value and high for high, i.e. value pricing
"Innovative drugs"	=	Any new drug, 85% of which are judged to add little therapeutic value
"Price controls"	=	Volume discounts to control prices by foreign countries
"Reimportation"	=	Global free trade made to sound like an unnatural act

Figure 6.3 A pharma lexicon.

Of special interest is the term "innovation." Pharmaceutical executives or their spokespersons emphasize that innovation is their noble contribution, and any reductions in revenues will reduce their ability to reduce suffering and death. But by "innovation" they mean any new product approved by the FDA, when in fact 65% of them are variations or new uses of existing molecules, and only about 35% of them are rated at the beginning of clinical trials to have the "potential" to offer a significant therapeutic benefit. But the old FDA rating system, before special interests forced it to be abandoned, used a more objective and differentiated scale that rated only about 2% of all new drugs as having the potential to offer an important therapeutic gain over existing drugs, and another 9% as offering a modest gain.[25] A leading independent European review came to the same conclusion after assessing the therapeutic value of every new drug that had come into use over the previous 22 years.[26]

This analysis may be regarded by some as biased against pharmaceutical firms, who, in reality, provide invaluable products and have thousands of dedicated employees full of integrity. But the evidence we read every month about unreported trials, undisclosed negative results, trials not designed using scientific criteria but designed to "prove" a new drug is statistically better than a sugar pill (the standard on which executives insist), fake ghost-written "scientific" articles, and misleading information to congressmen or citizens leaves no doubt that the bosses of these good employees have different values.

Pharmaceutical firms should make reasonable profits, but they should not siphon excess profits from every other company and impoverish patients. Any businessman who pays directly or indirectly for prescription drugs, or any public official charged with using taxpayers' hard-earned money efficiently, needs to ask why the most open, competitive market in pharmaceuticals in the world has consistently resulted in the highest prices? The much higher prices in the USA have spawned a consumer revolt and a growing number of internet channels for Americans to fill their prescriptions at half-price or less.[27] One response by GlaxoSmithKline was to cut off supplies to the participating Canadian pharmacies.[28] A critic observed, "Glaxo is not only compromising the health of the US patients who can only afford cheaper drugs, but is threatening the supply chain in Canada as a whole."

Stakeholder views of pricing

Prices are commercially constructed realities that most consumers take as facts. In a limited space, we shall focus on buyers and sellers, starting with the controlling party, the sellers.

The sellers' view of pricing

The true goal of corporate sellers such as pharmaceutical firms is to maximize revenues, profits, and growth. The goal is to charge as much as one can to each customer with as little competition as possible. Adam Smith understood this danger of greed and stipulated that there must be many informed rational buyers who can shop for value among many sellers, thus forcing them to compete among each other by lowering prices or increasing value. The result is like the market for laptop computers: their prices keep coming down as manufacturers keep making better ones to justify higher prices, which then begin to decline.

Contrast this with long-established markets for drugs to treat depression or pain or almost any major class. Prices on such older drugs keep being raised. A 1992 government report found, for example, that the price of Dilantin® increased 334% between 1985 and 1991, Tylenol® with codeine by 161%, Prolixin® by 113%, and Valium® by 109%.[29] The pharmaceutical industry insists that it raises prices little and that most of the cost increase comes from increased utilization. Industry-sponsored studies "prove" that this is so. Of course, in normal competitive markets, increased sales enable companies to reduce prices. Not surprisingly, studies external to the industry paint a different picture to the industry's claims. For example, Express Scripts is a large pharmacy benefit management company that tracks the expenses of its employer-clients closely, and its data support the Canadian data showing that drug companies increase prices on existing drugs more in the USA than in other countries and that these increases account for more than a third of overall cost increases.[30] The National Institute for Health Care Management Research and Education Foundation[31] also found that price increases accounted for more than a third of overall cost increases. Year after year, most of the new products offer no therapeutic gain but are given patent protection for monopoly pricing. Yet prices have risen substantially, not only on existing drugs but especially on the monopoly prices of new ones that physicians and patients are persuaded to substitute for the older and cheaper ones, even though they often provide little or no additional benefit.

How are such patterns of pricing possible? Pharmaceutical firms have succeeded in recruiting politicians and regulators to structure their markets so that they can control prices and maximize what they charge customers, with minimal downward pressure from competitors. The constructed reality of their markets has the following features.

Secret pricing and segmented markets

It might be called more politely "discretionary" or private pricing, but the reality was inadvertently revealed in John Hansen's[13] overview of US drug pricing. This was written for the medicines' project for the London School of Economics study on healthcare in major wealthy countries. He wrote: "Drug prices are established through arrangements between pharmaceutical manufacturers and a variety of private and public sector purchasers ..." "Arrangements" is not how one would describe normal markets; one does not buy one's laptop through an "arrange-ment." Essentially, the industry maintains that prices are proprietary information, a position that makes price competition impossible. The price depends on how much they want that customer's business, how large the order is, what seller rebates (or buyer kickbacks?) are part of the deal, what issues of market share are in play, to what extent the deal can be shaped to feature high-margin substitutes for low-margin ones, and so forth. Such practices contrast sharply from the principles of transparency, value for money, and consumer protection that characterize the price board in Canada and a number of other affluent, capitalist countries.[32]

Monopoly price protections

Patents, data exclusivity, and other pro-price regulations would take a book to describe, but a core point is that from the perspective of sellers, patents allow them to sell drugs at protected prices, and to raise these as they get older. Although the rationale for patents is to reward innovation and spur innovators to invent again by rewarding them with protection from price competition for a limited time, the realities diverge significantly from this original intent of the law. First, no one keeps track of how long it takes for drug companies to recover their R&D costs. The business plans for the large research-oriented firms are said to call for full recovery within five years, not 10 or 20. If patents were shorter, or proportional to how innovative a new drug is, it would spur companies to focus more on discovering breakthrough drugs and less on extending protection from normal competition.

The industry ceaselessly argues that high prices are a part of patents, that patents mean innovation, and that longer patents lead to more innovation. All three claims are false or untested. Patent law does not embody a right to a price or a profit, and most of the millions of patents never lead to any sale at all. The fortunate 5% (or less) find someone who will pay them something. Think of the inventors of all those patented parts in cell phones that nevertheless compete fiercely on price. Cell phone manufacturers paid them something, but not much or the cost of cell phones would be much higher. The claim that longer patents engender more innovation is untested because companies want it to remain untested, and logically it is absurd. It would mean that as patent length increased to 30, 50, or 100 years, we would be awash with innovation. But long patent protection from the spur of price competition *reduces* the need or desire to innovate and increases the focus on further patent protections.

Patents could be restructured to come closer to their societal goal of rewarding creativity without burdening society, while also fostering further innovation by exposing inventors, once again, to open price competition. For this reason generics are a vital contributor to innovation.

Any business model supports the view that new products make it or fail within a short time, exceptions notwithstanding. In pharmaceuticals, most patents are for details of manufacturing or administration or new uses, not for better active ingredients. Patents inhibit innovation. The patent system in now regarded, even by hard-core capitalist advocates, as a major impediment to innovation and economic growth. Pharmaceutical firms, however, fiercely defend patents as essential for getting back their R&D costs, and "globalization" centers heavily on imposing the longest and most restrictive patent-thicket strategies in the USA on the rest of the world so that monopoly prices will be paid in every part of the globe.

Company "rebates"

The rebates passed to wholesalers for promoting high-profit products are like the old, outlawed practice of kickback fees from the early twentieth century that can now put a physician in jail. Company rebates can work as a form of co-opting the agents of buyers and making them agents of the sellers.

There are related kinds of rebates, such as: small "grants" to physicians for prescribing more of a brand-name, expensive product; generous payments to physicians for recruiting patients to a trial; or handsome speaker fees for leading a continuing medical education course. Most worrisome are "research expenses" to leading specialists for participating in a Phase III trial and making them part of the research team. These costs are fully tax-deductible and may qualify for one of the research tax credits. These specialists will be paid $1000–$2000 to give a talk to colleagues about how the new drug works, or the nature of the clinical problem and how the new drug fits into a therapeutic response. They become promoters, essentially insider sales people, who give talks and write testimonials about the wonders of the new drug to colleagues at their academic health centers and the surrounding regional markets, where their colleagues regard them as leaders of their field. With the clinical experts signed up and paid off, payers – governments and employers – will find themselves paying for new drugs instead of old, like Vioxx rather than ibuprofen, at 100 times the price.

Brand loyalty

Another major pricing strategy with which we are all familiar. Drawing on decades of academic research on the psychology of advertising, Ralph Lauren, Prahda, and Pfizer each persuade users to prefer or insist on their brand products so that a higher price can be warranted because it is no longer competing against other choices. With drugs, free samples play a key role in brand loyalty because you do not want to change from the drug you have been taking during the critical initial period of treatment. (What might happen if your doctor switched you to a generic? Is it really the same?) The competition is over before it begins. To lock in still more sales, some companies have been found to offer illegal kickback schemes in which specialists can buy the drugs at low prices, bill Medicare at a much higher level, and pocket the difference.

Brand loyalty is very expensive to develop and nurture; only the big players can afford to try. No other business pours so much money into having attractive sales reps, highly trained in the arts of persuasion, visit market-makers (i.e. physicians) to tell them about the fine qualities of their most profitable drugs and to leave plenty of free samples that help get patients going on the drugs, thus assuring repeat sales for months or years to come. Brand loyalty increases prices twice over, once to pay for the high cost of establishing it, and again for the premium it commands. Neither has anything to do with more effective treatment but everything to do with market share and profits.

Market expansion

A great success story of modern marketing took the sneakers of the 1950s that were used only for sports and persuaded people to wear restyled versions all the time – to work, to parties, even to church. Large pharmaceutical firms do the same, despite very strict attention to exactly what the FDA approves drugs for and strict prohibitions against marketing for any other use. But the loophole as large as the clinical imagination is that physicians are permitted to try a drug for off-label uses. Big pharma is happy to fund nonrigorous clinical experiments by any physician who has an idea of how their drugs might be used on another condition, to pay again for a science writer to author the results, again for putting the results in the hands of every relevant physician, and again for having the enthusiastic off-label advocates promote their ideas. It is much cheaper, quicker, and more effective than conducting rigorous trials for FDA approval for the new, alleged uses. This circumvention of the FDA system is a major source of market expansion and increasing costs to governments and employers. It also undermines the goal of evidence-based medicine and the scientific credibility of physicians, as they take money to promote off-label use, which the FDA prohibits companies from mentioning themselves.

Another major form of market expansion focuses on getting people with mild or transient versions of real medical problems to take drugs. Still better is to market it for feeling better than good, to create a Prozac nation. Yet most of the DSM IV diagnostic terms lack any scientific basis,[33] and most new antidepressants are only marginally effective while also being addictive.[34,35]

A third form of market expansion involves taking health problems that can and should be addressed through nonpharmaceutical means and then getting people to think of pills as the solution to them. Examples include obesity, hypertension, mild diabetes, many respiratory problems, sleeping problems, and many sexual problems.[36]

A major new forum for market expansion is direct-to-consumer advertising. It undermines the whole basis of the system in which board-certified physicians, who have rigorous training, decide which patients need which controlled substance. Direct advertisements are a seller's dream and a payer's nightmare. Adverts seem to turn physicians into waiters: "Waiter, give me an Absolut martini." "Doctor, give me Nexium."

These four forms of market expansion account for most of the long-term volume growth, while turning out new variations ("me-too" drugs) under patent protection accounts for most of the short-term increase in revenues.[37] The goal is to have everyone under 40 taking two or three drugs regularly and everyone over 60 taking five to seven. The premise behind an industry-sponsored report that has been promoted throughout Europe and the USA is that the more drugs you take, the healthier you will be.[38]

Market creation

This is the complement to market expansion; it establishes entirely new "needs." Conrad and Leiter[39] trace the corporate construction of widespread erectile dysfunction, social anxiety disorder and generalized anxiety disorder, and extension of short stature to "normal shortness." Medawar and Hardon[35] provide a closely documented account of how drug companies have expanded "mental illness" and promoted ineffective or dangerous drugs for them. Hartley[36] describes how drug companies are creating "female sexual disorders" as a new "medical problem," replete with symposia led by leading clinical advocates, educational materials, and articles in the mass media, so that a demand is created in potential patients while clinicians gain a new readiness to dispense the treatment, even before drugs exist to treat the supposed problem. Thus, once companies have drugs to offer, the "need" for it, the new language for the "disease," and its norms of behavior and response will be established.

The buyers' view of pricing

If the principal goal of pharmaceutical companies is to maximize revenues, profits, and growth, the principal goal of buyers is to buy effective medicines at the lowest price. Since one party prescribes, another consumes, and a third often pays, the buyer's interests are conflated with those of the doctor and patient. Neither usually knows the prices of the drugs they are prescribing or ingesting, and if a health plan or insurer is paying all or most of the bill, they do not care. Yet in the end, it is taxpayers or patients who pay through their taxes or premiums, or in the form of reduced wages. Even when the patient does know the prices, as do the 70 million who have to pay cash because they have no insurance coverage for drugs, they are in no position to bargain.

Buyers are often less organized and concentrated than sellers, even when an entire country has a single price commission. Buyers are also more conflicted, confused, or ambivalent about their goals. For example, many countries want to hold down their rising bill for drugs, but they also want to help drug companies grow. States are no different, and they compete against one another in bestowing tax concessions and special benefits on pharmaceutical companies to set up operations in Minnesota, or Pennsylvania, or shall it be Alabama? The UK is unique in having it both ways. It supports a thriving pharmaceutical sector by rewarding discoveries of new molecules (but not derivative variations) and by guaranteeing profits within a generous range, but it also limits what companies can charge their health system. What they charge other countries, like the USA, is their own business. Thus they get costs reasonable for their own system while supporting a thriving industry. By contrast, the USA rewards derivative research as richly as it does breakthrough research, and it lets companies charge what they want, including regular price increases, to a fragmented field of buyers.

US buyers who are serious about getting lower prices, such as many state Medicaid programs, many insurers, managed care plans, and employers, cannot control most of the major causes of increased expenditures that were described above. Further, only a few have the expertise to tackle drug costs. The large drug companies have spent years structuring markets to block or frustrate the goal of buying effective medicine at the lowest prices.

The consumer revolt against high prices

After years of enduring world-high prices, Americans began to revolt against them in the late 1990s.[27] Begun by senior citizens' groups in Maine, Vermont, and other border states it became by 2000 the primary election topic that all candidates had to address. The movement has grown vertically into well-funded institutionalized forms, such as a governors' association to bring down prices, a coalition of large employers to do the same, the dedication of foundations to fund price-lowering initiatives, and the formal amalgamation of grassroots organizations into national consortia that have mounted large class-action lawsuits against most of the major companies for improperly extending monopoly prices and thus causing extensive pain, suffering, and financial hardship to millions of sick Americans.[40]

The major firms have responded by taking to court every effort to lower prices. If they lose, they appeal until they wear down the opposition, just as the tobacco companies did for decades. In the USA, at least, they are also creating pseudo-grassroots organizations and hire lobbying firms to write grassroots letters and petitions. These counter-movements appear to confound or neutralize legislative efforts to get lower prices; but it is not a very comfortable position to have national consortia of citizens' groups taking one to court on behalf of millions of patients,[39] large employers opposing one's pricing policies, and more than three dozen governors and state legislatures bent on imposing lower prices and generic substitution for their state programs. These organized buyers are changing the balance of power in pharmaceutical markets and the prices that companies get. The coming decade should be lively.

References

1 Productivity Commission of Australia (2001) *International Pharmaceutical Price Differences: research report.* Productivity Commission of Australia, Melbourne.

2 (2005) Communications reported on ip-health-admin@lists-essential.org, October 24, and thereafter.

3 Pollack A (2005) Is a bird flu drug really so vexing? *New York Times.* 5 November: C1, C13.

4 Wall Street Journal (2001) Senate panel approves a bill on delays for generic drugs. *Wall Street Journal,* October 19: A16.

5 Harris G (2001) Bayer is accused of profiteering on Cipro. *Wall Street Journal.* 26 October: A6.

6 Carroll J and Winslow R (2001) Bayer agrees to slash prices for Cipro drug. *Wall Street Journal.* October 25.

7 Vedantam S (2001) HHS's varying costs for Cipro criticized. *Washington Post.* October 26.

8 Socolar D and Sager A (2002) *Windfall Profits Despite Discounted Prices: small manufacturing cost for Cipro yields estimated $70 million windfall.* Health Reform Program, Boston University School of Public Health, Boston.

9 Libby J, Kataiz RS, McCubbrey JB, Becker RD and Cohen N (2002) *AIDS Healthcare Foundation vs Glaxosmithkline.* Los Angeles: US Central District Court of California, Los Angeles.

10 Families USA (2003) *Out of Bounds: rising prescription drug prices for seniors.* Families USA, Washington, DC.

11 Families USA (2004) *Sticker Shock: rising prescription drug prices for seniors.* Families USA, Washington, DC.

12 Gross DJ, Schondelmeyer SW and Raetzman SO (2004) *Trends in Manufacturer Prices of Brand Name Prescription Drugs Used by Older Americans, 2000 through 2003.* AARP Public Policy Institute, Washington, DC.

13 Hansen J (2002) *Country Profile: United States: prescription drug pricing and reimbursement policy.* LSE Study on Healthcare in Individual Countries, London, G10 Medicines.

14 Cantor DJ (1998) *CRS Report for Congress – Prescription Drugs: factors influencing their pricing.* Congressional Research Service, Washington, DC.

15 Patented Medicine Prices Review Board (2002) *Annual Report 2001.* Patented Medicine Prices Review Board, Ottowa.

16 Mrazek MF (2002) Comparative approaches to pharmaceutical price regulation in the European Union. *Croat Med J.* **43**: 453–61.

17 Elgie RG (2001) *A Delicate Balance – Can Governments Promote R&D and Control Drug Costs at the Same Time?* Patented Medicine Prices Review Board, Toronto.

18 Gregson N, Sparrowhawk K, Mauskopf J and Paul J (2005) Pricing medicines: theory and practice, challenges and opportunities. *Nat Rev Drug Discov.* **4**: 121–30.

19 Light DW (2004) Interview with FM Scherer. September, 13.

20 DiMasi JA, Hansen RW and Grabowski H (2003) The price of innovation: new estimates of drug development costs. *J Health Econ.* **22**: 151–85.

21 Light DW and Warburton RN (2005) Extraordinary claims require extraordinary evidence. *J Health Econ.* **24**: 1030–3.

22 DiMasi JA, Hansen RW and Grabowski HG (2005) Reply: extraordinary claims require extraordinary evidence. *J Health Econ.* **24**: 1034–44.

23 Light DW and Lexchin J (2005) Foreign free riders and the high price of US medicines. *BMJ.* **331**: 958–60.

24 Goozner M (2004) *The $800 Million Pill: the truth behind the cost of new drugs.* University of California Press, Berkeley, CA.

25 US Senate Select Committee on Small Business (1979) *Competitive Problems in the Drug Industry*. US Government Publications Office, Washington, DC.

26 Prescrire International (2003) A review of new drugs and indications in 2002: financial speculation or better patient care? *Prescrire Int.* **12**: 74–7.

27 Light DW, Castellblanch R, Arrendondo P and Socolar D (2003) No exit and the organization of voice in biotechnology and pharmaceuticals. *J Health Polit Policy Law.* **28**: 473–507.

28 Dyer G (2003) Drugs group threat to Canada. *Financial Times*, January 14: 2.

29 General Accounting Office (1992) *Prescription Drugs: changes in prices for selected drugs*. GAO, Washington, DC.

30 Express Scripts (annual) *Drug Trend Report*. Express Scripts, St Louis.

31 National Institute for Health Care Management Research and Educational Foundation (2002) *Prescription Drug Expenditures in 2001: another year of escalating costs*. NIHCM, Washington, DC. Available from www.nihcm.org (accessed June 3, 2006).

32 Elgie RG (2002) *How the Patented Medicine Prices Review Board Contributes to Controlling Drug Prices in Canada*. Patented Medicine Prices Review Board, Toronto.

33 Horwitz A (2001) *Creating Mental Illness*. University of Chicago Press, Chicago, IL.

34 Healy D (1997) *The Anti-depressant Era*. Harvard University Press, Cambridge, MA.

35 Medawar C and Hardon A (2004) *Medicines Out of Control?* Aksant, London.

36 Hartley H (2003) "Big Pharma" in our bedrooms: an analysis of the medicalization of women's sexual problems. *Advances Gender Res.* **7**: 89–129.

37 Morgan SG, Bassett KL, Wright JM *et al.* (2005) 'Breakthrough' drugs and growth in expenditure on prescription drugs in Canada. *BMJ.* **331**: 815–6.

38 Gilbert J and Rosenberg P (2004) *Addressing the Innovation Divide: imbalance innovation*. Bain & Company, Boston, MA.

39 Conrad P and Leiter V (2004) Medicalization, markets and consumers. *J Health Soc Behav.* **45** (Suppl): 158–76.

40 Prescription Access Litigation Project (2003–2005) Information available from www.communitycatalyst.org (accessed November 26, 2005).

Chapter 7

Potential savings from therapeutic substitution of 10 of Canada's most dispensed prescription drugs

Alan Cassels and Joel Lexchin

Background

Although many drugs may be effective at controlling symptoms and reducing hospitalizations, the mounting cost of new medicines and the growing portion of our healthcare dollars needed to pay for them will force decision makers at all levels – payer, prescriber, and patient – to act in ways that are increasingly more rational and prudent.

Any discussion on comparative cost-effectiveness of pharmaceutical therapy should start with a definition as to what constitutes "rational" use of drugs. The 1985 World Health Organization Conference of Experts on the Rational Use of Drugs stated: "Rational use of drugs requires that patients receive medications appropriate to their clinical needs, in doses that meet their own individual requirements for an adequate period of time, and at the lowest cost to them and their community."[1]

This definition is accompanied by a description of appropriate prescribing which includes the following considerations: that a drug has been prescribed for an appropriate indication (its use is entirely based on medical rationale and the drug therapy prescribed is an effective and safe treatment for the indication); an appropriate drug has been chosen (based on an assessment of effectiveness, safety, and cost considerations); that the drug has been administered to an appropriate patient (no contraindications exist, the likelihood of adverse reactions is minimal, and the drug is acceptable to the patient); and the patient has been provided with relevant, accurate, and clear information regarding her or his condition and the medication(s) prescribed.[1]

It is clear that one way to improve appropriate prescribing is by designing and implementing prescribing guidelines for physicians. The actual use of these guidelines, however, shows that physicians are slow to adopt them. In a two-year study of an Edmonton primary care clinic only 23% of 969 patients received a first-line drug as recommended by Canadian guidelines.[2]

Of the key health conditions associated with the most heavily prescribed drugs, such as heartburn, high cholesterol, and high blood pressure, most treatment guidelines recommend that physicians start with a range of nonpharmacologic treatments. These sometimes obviate the need for a prescription in the first place and therefore prescribing a medication on a first presentation of nonsevere signs or symptoms is often inappropriate. With high blood pressure, for example, there is reasonable evidence that dietary modifications (including reducing salt intake) can help some patients achieve targeted levels of blood pressure control.[3]

Avoiding certain foods or alcohol can help alleviate symptoms of gastro-esophageal reflux disease (GERD) and those symptoms can sometimes be treated with over-the-counter (OTC) products. For patients with high cholesterol but no other risk factors for heart disease, the pharmacologic modification of cholesterol levels has a modest impact on morbidity and mortality (*see* Chapter 8). However, for most patients lifestyle changes and self-care therapies should be the first, and sometimes the only treatment recommended by a physician. And nonpharmacologic therapies have a growing body of evidence to support their use in a variety of other conditions. The evidence suggests that psychological interventions are at least as effective as pharmacotherapy in treating depression, even if severe, especially when patient-rated measures are used and long-term follow-up is considered.[4]

This chapter will add to current investigations around the extent to which Canada could reduce its overall drug expenditures by decreasing the use of expensive, heavily prescribed medications in favor of equally effective but less expensive alternatives.[5] We are putting a select group of pharmaceuticals under the microscope and asking: Are these drugs being prescribed without considering the comparative cost-effectiveness of a range of other products that are just as effective? While the information presented applies most specifically to Canada, the findings also apply to the USA and other countries.

Methods

We used a list, produced by IMS Canada, of the top 100 most-dispensed drugs in Canada in 2004. We cross-referenced that list with a list of the top-selling 250 products by dollar volume, paid for through private drug plans in Canada. This list was tabulated from claims processed from June to December 2004 by BCE Emergis, which is a prescription claims processing company that handles over 40% of the private drug claims in Canada.

From the BCE Emergis list we selected the top 10 brand-name drugs that were not available generically and for which independent reference sources identified a less costly alternative that was equally effective and safe in most instances. We used the IMS list to determine the number of prescriptions written annually in Canada for these products. To simplify calculations we assumed that all prescriptions were written for the defined daily dose (DDD). This is a concept developed by the Nordic Council on Medicines to study drug utilization. It is the assumed average maintenance dose per day for a drug used for its main indication in adults.[6]

We used two sources for prices: the main one was produced by BC Pharmacare, the public drug program in British Columbia (BC), which indicates the price of treatment based on the average prices paid for these products between January and June 2004. Where we couldn't find the prices in BC, we used Ontario prices. Previous work has established that prices for brand-name drugs are virtually uniform across Canada.[7]

To compute overall savings we used the difference in price of the DDD between the drug selected from the BCE Emergis list and its therapeutically equivalent comparator, multiplied that difference by 30 (assuming each prescription is for a

30-day period), and then multiplied by the annual number of prescriptions. We assumed that substituting a less costly drug would not be appropriate in every case and therefore calculated cost savings at two different levels of substitution, 100% and 25%, in order to provide a range of potential savings.

Findings

The drugs upon which this analysis is based are those that, based on price and volume of use, have the most significant impact on the budgets of drug plan payers and are among the most dispensed products in Canada. They include 10 separate prescription products which treat five main conditions, namely, hypertension, high cholesterol, acid reflux, arthritis, and depression. The drugs are:

- two cholesterol-lowering drugs: Lipitor® (atorvastatin) and Crestor® (rosuvastatin)
- three drugs for hypertension and angina: Altace® (ramipril), Norvasc® (amlodipine), and Adalat XL® (nifedipine)
- one anti-arthritis drug: Celebrex® (celecoxib)
- three drugs for acid reflux: Pantoloc® (pantoprazole), Nexium® (esomeprazole), and Losec® (omeprazole)
- one antidepressant: Effexor XR® (venlafaxine).

Table 7.1 lists the possible savings achieved by making 100% and 25% alternative choices for the 10 products. Our findings show that if physicians were able to achieve 100% substitution for each of these 10 top-selling drugs, they would engender drug budget savings of about $970 million, or about 45% of the costs of these drugs. This could be achieved without compromising clinical outcomes. Even if only a quarter of doctors practiced therapeutic substitutions for these 10 drugs, Canada would reduce its drug bill by $242 million, or about 11% of the cost of these drugs. These savings need to be regarded as estimates since we only selected a single dose for each of the drugs and we assumed that all prescriptions were written for a 30-day period. Clearly, in the real world of prescribing these simplifications may not apply.

Below is a brief breakdown of the products on this "top 10" list and a less expensive, therapeutically equivalent comparator.

Lipitor (atorvastatin) and Crestor (rosuvastatin)

These are statins for the treatment of high cholesterol; annual script count: 9 753 000 and 1 909 000, respectively; savings range: $54 million to $219 million.

In 2003, according to IMS Health Canada, cholesterol-lowering medications were the fastest-growing class among the country's most heavily prescribed classes of medications.[8] The cholesterol-lowering drug Lipitor (atorvastatin) is the world's top-selling drug and holds first place in almost any prescription drug budget, yet, surprisingly, it is prescribed with no evidence of superiority in preventing heart attacks and strokes over other cholesterol-lowering agents. According to a recently published meta-analysis conducted by the Oregon Health Resources Commission, there is "good quality evidence for improved cardiac outcomes with Lipitor®, Lescol®, Mevacor®, Pravachol®, and Zocor® when compared with placebo," but there are "no studies which directly compare the efficacy of different statins in the

Table 7.1 Cost* savings if "top 10" brand-name drugs were substituted by cheaper, therapeutically equivalent drugs

Rank on "top 10" list	Brand name (generic name)	Cost per tablet of most-prescribed dose size (in BC)	IMS data on number of scripts†	Total cost (assuming all scripts written in that dose size)	Therapeutic equivalent	Cost per tablet of therapeutic equivalent	Total cost savings (assuming 100% substitution)	Total cost savings (assuming 25% substitution)
1	Lipitor (atorvastatin)	1.73	9 753 000	506 180 700	pravastatin	0.98	219 442 500	54 860 625
2	Effexor XR (venlafaxine)	1.65	4 441 000	219 829 000	fluoxetine	1.01	85 267 200	21 316 800
3	Altace (ramipril)	1.23	7 381 000	171 358 900	lisinopril	0.84	86 357 700	21 589 425
4	Losec (omeprazole)	2.57	3 682 000	283 882 200	Pariet® (rabeprazole)	1.41	128 133 600	32 033 400
5	Norvasc (amlodipine)	1.46	4 889 000	214 138 200	generic hydro-chlorothiazide	0.01	212 671 500	53 167 875
6	Celebrex (celecoxib)	2.39	3 030 000	217 251 000	naproxen	1.47	83 628 000	20 907 000
7	Pantaloc (pantoprazole)	2.14	3 380 000	216 996 000	Pariet (rabeprazole)	1.41	74 022 000	18 505 500
8	Adalat XL (nifedipine)	0.52	2 590 000	40 404 000	generic hydro-chlorothiazide	0.01	39 627 000	9 906 750
9	Nexium (esomeprazole)	2.24	1 673 000	112 425 600	Pariet (rabeprazole)	1.41	41 657 700	10 414 425
10	Crestor (rosuvastatin)	1.42	1 909 000	81 323 400	pravastatin	0.98	25 198 800	6 299 700
Total				2 164 789 000			970 807 200	242 701 800

BC, British Colombia.

* All costs are in Canadian dollars and are based on prices in British Colombia.

† Sales figures refer to the whole of Canada for 2004.

reduction of cardiovascular events."[9] A recent Canadian study confirmed that statins are equally effective for secondary prevention in elderly patients after a myocardial infarction.[10]

It would be safe to say that in the absence of evidence of superiority of Lipitor, then physicians should be prescribing the cheapest effective dose of any of the statins. We chose generic pravastatin at a DDD of 20 mg.

Altace (ramipril)

This is an angiotensin-converting enzyme (ACE) inhibitor for the treatment of hypertension; annual script count: 7 381 000; savings range: $21 million to $86 million.

ACE inhibitors can be used for a variety of indications, including hypertension, congestive heart failure, and myocardial infarction. In uncomplicated hypertension, initial treatment with diuretics is considered most appropriate but because of the multiplicity of uses of ACE inhibitors we have limited our choice of comparators to other drugs in the same class. Although some ACE inhibitors have indications that others do not have, in general it is believed that there is a class effect such that at appropriate doses all drugs in this class are equally safe and effective.[11,12] The alternative that we selected for Altace is generic lisinopril at a DDD of 10 mg.

Norvasc (amlodipine) and Adalat XL (nifedipine)

These are calcium channel blockers (CCBs) for the treatment of hypertension; annual script count: 4 889 000 and 2 590 000, respectively; savings range: $53 million to $212 million.

For hypertension or high blood pressure, CCBs, such as Norvasc (amlodipine) and Adalat (nifedipine), are widely prescribed despite the fact that the evidence on treating uncomplicated hypertension suggests that, at best, this class of drugs should be a physician's third or fourth choice after (and in order) diuretics, beta-blockers, and ACE inhibitors, all of which are less expensive. According to IMS Health Canada data, the most frequently prescribed drugs for hypertension are (in order) ACE inhibitors, CCBs, and angiotensin receptor blockers, which together make up 78% of all antihypertensive prescriptions written. Diuretics make up only 18%.[13]

CCBs are prescribed for the treatment of angina, alone or in combination with hypertension. In these cases substitution with a diuretic would not be appropriate. However, hypertension is the largest therapeutic subcategory in cardiovascular disease and therefore, in the majority of cases, diuretics are the most rational first choice, and more use would generate significant savings. Using the most effective and safest agent, simple diuretics, a physician could treat 200 hypertensive patients for the price of one treated with CCBs.[14]

Additionally, the symptoms attributable to thiazides, beta-blockers, and CCBs were strongly dose-related, and combining low-dose drug treatment has been shown to increase efficacy and reduce adverse effects.[15] The alternative that we chose was generic hydrochlorothiazide at a DDD of 25 mg.

Celebrex (celecoxib)

This is a selective nonsteroidal anti-inflammatory drug for the treatment of inflammation and pain that accompanies arthritis. Annual script count: 3 030 000; savings range $20 million to $83 million.

For pain and inflammation due to arthritis, evidence shows that the newer COX-2 selective nonsteroidal anti-inflammatory drugs (NSAIDs), such as Celebrex and Vioxx, are not superior to the class of over 25 nonselective NSAIDs.

The Oregon Health Resources Commission NSAIDs Subcommittee Report agreed by consensus that "evidence comparing celecoxib and rofecoxib is inconsistent and inconclusive and there were no comparison studies including valdecoxib. Current evidence does not support the conclusion that there are differences in either efficacy or safety among COX-2 inhibitors."[16]

The Commission found 10 trials comparing celecoxib and nonselective NSAIDs. Not all had been fully published in peer-reviewed literature. Two trials found celecoxib and naproxen to be equally effective. An unpublished trial, raising the concern of publication bias, found naproxen to be superior. The Commission's key conclusion was: "The subcommittee agrees by consensus that evidence does not demonstrate any difference in efficacy among nonselective NSAIDS, COX-2 preferential NSAIDs and COX-2 inhibitors."[16]

Some may argue that it is inappropriate to limit the range of NSAIDs available to patients. In a study of a prior authorization scheme affecting NSAIDs, physicians were limited in prescribing to a specified set of NSAIDS yet this limitation showed no impact on health status.[17]

In sum, since some patients might respond to any NSAID, and it is impossible to predict how any person will respond to any NSAID, if the doctor prescribes one, they should probably consider ASA (aspirin) or acetaminophen (Tylenol®), which are available over the counter, or if a prescription is required, low-dose naproxen or ibuprofen. The alternative that we chose was a prescription-only drug, generic naproxen at a DDD of 0.5 mg.

Pantaloc (pantoprazole), Nexium (esomeprazole), and Losec (omeprazole)

These are proton pump inhibitors (PPIs) for the treatment of peptic ulcers and heartburn; annual script count: 3 380 000, 1 673 000, and 3 682 000, respectively; savings range: $61 million to $244 million.

Typical treatment for patients with mild to moderate symptoms of heartburn, or gastro-esophageal reflux disease (GERD), starts with simple lifestyle changes (diet, exercise, timing of meals, etc.) and then antacids. If antacids are not effective, patients can move to H2-blockers, such as cimetidine (Tagamet®), ranitidine (Zantac®), nizatidine (Axid®), or famotidine (Pepcid®), which work by reducing the amount of acid in the stomach.

PPIs, such as Losec, Nexium, and Pantoloc, are first-line therapy in refractory cases of esophagitis or for severe erosive esophagitis. In addition, PPIs in combination with selected antibiotics are drugs of choice for curative therapy for duodenal ulcers. Although PPIs, which make up three of the 10 drugs, are second-line treatment after failure of lifestyle alterations or H2-blockers, because they can be first-line in other cases, we have limited our choice of comparators to other PPIs only.

All five PPIs on the market are equally effective at equivalent doses; no trials have demonstrated an intrinsic therapeutic advantage of the newest PPI, Nexium, over other PPIs at equivalent doses. The initial choice of agent should therefore depend on cost. In Canada, the PPIs Pariet and Apo-Omeprazole® represent a reduction in cost of approximately 40% over other PPI drugs. We have used as a comparator a DDD of 20 mg of rabeprazole (Pariet) which is priced almost exactly at the generic price of omeprazole.

Effexor XR (venlafaxine)

This is a serotonin and norepinephrine reuptake inhibitor (SNRI) for the treatment of depression; annual script count: 4 441 000; savings range: $21 million to $85 million.

According to Uhegarty et al.[18] all antidepressants have equal efficacy in the treatment of major depression. It is therefore the adverse effect profile which largely determines the choice of antidepressant for this condition.

A large majority of American and Canadian psychiatrists and family physicians favor either the SNRI or SSRI (e.g. Prozac, Paxil, or Zoloft) classes of antidepressants as "first-line" medications. An older class of antidepressants, the tricyclics (TCAs), are equivalent to the SNRIs and SSRIs in effectiveness and are less expensive; however, SNRIs and SSRIs may be viewed more favorably by physicians than the TCAs because of their relative safety in overdose.

There are few compelling reasons to pick a SNRI over an SSRI (or vice versa) for treatment of uncomplicated major depression.[19] While the side effect profile of Effexor XR may occasionally make it a first-line agent, in the majority of cases there is no reason not to initially choose generic fluoxetine at a DDD of 20 mg.

Discussion

Prescribing and payment decisions need to be "evidence-based," that is, based on objective, quality scientific research concerning benefits, harms, convenience, and cost-effectiveness of competing treatments. Even though the body of available evidence supporting rational pharmaceutical use is growing, prescription drugs are still often used irrationally: in the wrong patients for the wrong reasons; using more expensive agents when cheaper ones are equally effective; and in instances where harm likely exceeds benefit. The potential for massive waste is staggering. According to some estimates almost half of the elderly experience at least one episode of questionable prescribing every year. Although it is difficult to be sure exactly what the costs are of this inappropriate prescribing, it is highly likely that they are substantial.[20]

Why are doctors writing prescriptions for costly drugs when there are less expensive products that are equally effective and safe? To begin with, doctors frequently do not take cost into consideration when prescribing. Even when they do, there is good evidence that for the most part they are unaware of the cost of drugs, either in absolute terms (how much individual drugs cost) or in relative terms (what different drugs cost in relation to one another).[21,22]

In part, this lack of knowledge can be ascribed to the fact that doctors are not the ones who either sell or buy the drugs that they prescribe. However, this is far from the whole story; a major factor is where doctors get their information from. The pharmaceutical companies' people seem to be highly effective in influencing doctors' prescribing behavior, a subject that was explored in Chapter 5. Furthermore, questionnaires filled out by doctors who have seen sales representatives, and audiotapes of interactions between these two groups, reveal that the price of medications is rarely mentioned.[23,24]

Even doctors who rely on guidelines to aid their prescribing may sometimes be receiving biased information. The cost of guidelines is often underwritten by pharmaceutical companies and authors frequently have financial relationships with the companies whose products are mentioned. Moreover, these conflicts of interest are usually not reported in the guidelines.[25,26] This problem was discussed in Chapter 3.

New drugs are generally the most heavily promoted, and these tend to be more expensive. In Canada, companies are spending an estimated $2.1 billion dollars per year on promotion. In 2000, less than one year after Vioxx appeared on the market, Merck spent over $6 million on its promotion, buying over 1000 pages in medical journals, sending sales representatives to doctors' offices almost 50 000 times, and leaving behind over one million pills.[27]

The combined forces of industry-influenced guidelines and promotion can be seen in prescribing patterns for high blood pressure medications and anti-inflammatory drugs. In the 1980s and 1990s CCBs and ACE inhibitors were replacing diuretics as first-line therapy for hypertension. While there were theoretical grounds for believing that these drugs might be better, there was no actual clinical evidence in the form of morbidity and mortality data. In fact, only the diuretics had been shown to reduce the risk of heart attacks and strokes. In a Canadian study, the percentage of patients receiving diuretics fell, between 1985 and 1995, from 31% to 17%, while the percentage given CCBs and ACE inhibitors went from 2% to 20% and from 5% to 25%, respectively.[28] These changes occurred despite the huge difference in prices; diuretics cost 5–10 cents per day while prices for the other two classes were around $1 per day. Helping to fuel this change were guidelines on the treatment of hypertension from presumably authoritative bodies like the World Health Organization. When its guidelines were released in 1999, they were strongly criticized for their heavy reliance on a small number of studies sponsored by the drug industry. All but one of the 18 members of the committee that drafted the guidelines had financial ties to drug companies that made either CCBs or ACE inhibitors.[29] The ALLHAT study, published in 2002, compared different classes of antihypertensive agents and was financed by the US National Heart, Lung and Blood Institute. It reaffirmed that diuretics were superior to the other classes in preventing some of the consequences of hypertension and recommended that they should be the preferred first-step antihypertensive therapy.[30]

Both Vioxx and Celebrex, collectively known as COX-2 inhibitors, were introduced to the Canadian market in 1999 as anti-inflammatory medications that were supposed to cause fewer gastrointestinal side effects than traditional anti-inflammatory drugs (NSAIDs). However, there was never any evidence establishing this fact for Celebrex and the overall safety profile of Vioxx was in doubt from shortly after its launch. The volume of promotion for Vioxx was described earlier. Celebrex was close behind with over $6 million spent on promotion, 77 000 visits by sales representatives, and just shy of one million samples being left behind.[27]

A supplement in the fall 2000 issue of the *Canadian Journal of Clinical Pharmacology* recommended the use of COX-2 medications as first-line therapy in the treatment of rheumatoid arthritis and osteoarthritis.[31] These guidelines were titled "evidence-based" to give them additional weight. Although the front of the supplement states that it was funded through unrestricted education grants from Searle and Pfizer, there was no mention made of whether these two companies funded the consensus conference itself. There was also no statement about whether the authors or any of the other participants in the conference had any relationships with these two companies. Once again, there was a large price discrepancy between these two new products and older NSAIDs, the former costing over $1 per day and some of the latter being 5–10 cents a day. By 2002, even with the lack of evidence for safety and the large price premium, in some Canadians provinces 66% to 70% of all prescriptions for NSAIDs were for COX-2s, and this class of drugs accounted for about 85% of all spending on NSAIDs.[32] The subsequent fate of Vioxx is well known (*see* Chapter 4), being pulled from the market in the fall of 2004 because of its association with a significant increase in cardiovascular disease.

The rapid increase in the use of more expensive medications highlights the main limitation in the ability of the Patented Medicine Prices Review Board (PMPRB) to control drug expenditures in Canada. The PMPRB was established in 1987 to protect consumer interests with powers to limit the introductory prices for new patented drugs and prevent prices for existing patented drugs from rising by more than the rate of inflation. Within this context the PMPRB has been a success: between 1988 and 2000 the rate of inflation for the price of patented medications rose by just 0.5% per year.[33] International comparisons also indicate success: the ratio of Canadian prices to those in seven other countries (France, Germany, Italy, Sweden, Switzerland, the UK, USA) has dropped from 1.23 in 1987 to just 0.95 in 2003.[33] However, the PMPRB has no control over physician prescribing decisions and therefore cannot prevent doctors from substituting newer, more expensive medications for older ones that are less expensive but no less safe or effective. The findings that we presented earlier attest to the magnitude of this problem. At the level of the individual prescription, on average, between 1997 and 2001 the cost of a prescription for nonpatented medications (read older, less expensive) increased 2.3% annually to $22.94. In stark contrast, during the same period patented medications (read newer, more expensive) went up by 6.2% annually to a cost of $84.36.[11]

The problem with using more expensive drugs when less costly ones will work just as well needs to be tackled at a couple of levels. From the perspective of government policy the Reference Drug Program (as described in Chapter 15) or maximum allowable cost (MAC) are policy options in use in Canadian provinces. Under Reference Pricing, drugs in the same class judged "therapeutically equivalent" are priced at the least cost "reference" price and the provincial plan pays for the treatment at that level. This encourages physicians to prescribe, and patients to take, drugs that at least initially are the most cost-effective drug in the class.[34]

Experience with Reference Pricing and other cost-saving programs suggests that price incentives alone have a limited ability to change prescribing patterns and to lower overall costs, especially among the elderly. Soumerai and coworkers[35] have demonstrated that in the absence of physician education programs, administrative decisions at the policy level will have variable effects, not all of them positive.

The most effective efforts at physician education are likely to involve multiple programs that build upon each other for effectiveness. In Australia, Roughead et al.[36] showed that it was possible to decrease prescribing of a dangerous antibiotic through a combination of regulatory interventions, warnings in drug bulletins, medical journal articles, and changes in antibiotic guidelines. Closer to home, teleconferences, small group workshops, and articles in drug bulletins were used in British Columbia to change prescribing for hypertension in favor of first-line agents.[37]

Drug plan managers and the medical community at large should see it as a priority to use the existing evidence to construct independent evidence-based prescribing guidelines and to institute other management tools, such as academic detailing, that provide comparative information for conditions that commonly result in pharmacotherapy.[38]

The Oregon Health Resources Commission[39] provides a model on how to achieve consensus around the concepts we are proposing. In 2000, it spent nine months holding public meetings, hearing testimony from consumer groups, the pharmaceutical industry, pharmacists, doctors, patient advocates, state employees, and others, and reviewed hundreds of articles from peer-reviewed journals. The recommendations of the Commission are particularly cogent. They concluded that the best model to control prescription drug costs while improving access to pharmaceuticals was by developing a statewide evidence-based formulary. They recommended a process be established which examines "available medical, social, and economic evidence from both a technical and policy perspective, in order to estimate the cost effectiveness of pharmaceuticals relative to alternatives."[37] The emphasis on basing recommendations on quality evidence is unarguable, and the importance of proving cost-effectiveness should be a model worthy of replication in other jurisdictions. Since holding its hearings it has gone on to establish the Oregon Drug Effectiveness Review Project which, during its three-year lifespan (2003–2006), will produce evidence-based guidelines on the use of 25 different drug classes.

Additional factors to consider

Any study on cost comparisons is obviously dependent on the vagaries of the data sources used. The composition of any list is time-limited and somewhat jurisdiction-limited. Differences in factors such as prescribing patterns, marketing campaigns, and formulary restrictions will affect which drugs make it to a list such as the one we have constructed, yet the general principles of therapeutic substitution still apply. The fact is, in whatever jurisdiction is chosen, there will be a range of prices for comparable, therapeutically equivalent products, be they lower-priced brand name products or generic drugs. When looking at generic substitution, other factors come into play, such as the fact that patents expire at different times in different jurisdictions and the launch of generic versions varies by jurisdiction. All these factors affect the cost of the replacement drugs used in these calculations.

The cost of educating physicians and patients would be an important part of enacting policies to encourage people to use more cost-effective drugs, and educational programs alone may be of limited effect. What is also not considered here are the costs of switching or further costs of adjudication, implementing special authority or prior authorization, or putting programs in place to communicate with physicians and patients.

Data on the rate of rational prescribing would need to be gathered before implementing a switching policy in order to estimate possible savings and the costs involved in instituting a program of therapeutic substitution. This would include knowing with better precision the level of inappropriate prescribing in each category, costs associated with that prescribing, the proportion of patients that are being prescribed these drugs first-line, as opposed to second- or third-line, and the proportion of beneficiaries who have diagnostically proven conditions that justify pharmaceutical therapy.

Conclusions

The overall role of pharmaceuticals in healthcare is undisputed but that does not mean drugs should ever be overused, or misused, and certainly not where clinically neutral changes in prescribing can result in such enormous savings to the healthcare system.

Older drugs sometimes represent tremendous value in comparison to newer drugs, yet their value is often not marketed to physicians because these are often generic products that yield low profits. Physicians need access to unbiased information that compares drugs in terms of their effectiveness, safety, and costs in the form of clear, evidence-based formularies that they can incorporate into their practice.

The need to push for better and more appropriate use of drugs in the healthcare system is growing in urgency, not only because of financial concerns but also because of the vast opportunities at hand to use available evidence to improve the quality of pharmaceutical care for patients. As drug costs escalate, the gap between medical need and the ability to pay for medicines prescribed by doctors will only grow.

The data presented here demonstrate the enormous level of savings that could be achieved with better and more cost-effective prescribing. It will hopefully focus much more attention on actions required to achieve better and more cost-effective use of pharmaceuticals, and better physician education around comparative cost-effectiveness of competing products. While the data on which this study is based come from Canada, there is little doubt that a similar situation exists in the USA and other Western countries.

While this study only deals with the top 10 drugs in terms of budgetary impact, which represent $2.2 billion of the entire $18 billion Canadians spent in 2004 on prescription drugs,[40] the principles of therapeutic substitution could be applied to the entire body of prescribed medicines. It is possible that making simple substitutions for most of the highest-cost pharmaceuticals could also result in many billions more in savings. These findings not only apply internationally with reference to any nation's top-selling drugs but also to most drugs on a drug plan's formulary for which there are often therapeutically equivalent and less expensive alternatives from which physicians may choose.

References

1 Laing R, Hogerzeil H and Ross-Degnan D (2001) Ten recommendations to improve use of medicines in developing countries. *Health Policy Plan.* **16**: 13–20. Available from: http://dcc2.bumc.bu.edu/prdu/Trainers_Guides/acknowledgements.htm (accessed March 14, 2004).

2 McAlister FA, Teo KK, Lewanczuk RZ, Wells G and Montague TJ (1997) Contemporary practice patterns in the management of newly diagnosed hypertension. *Can Med Assoc J.* **157**: 23–30.

3 Charlton KE (2006) Diet and blood pressure: moving beyond preoccupation with salt to composite dietary patterns. In: Temple NJ, Wilson T and Jacobs DR, eds. *Nutritional Health: strategies for disease prevention* (2e). Humana Press, Totowa, NJ.

4 Antonuccio DO, Danton WG, DeNelsky GY, Greenberg RP and Gordon JS (1999) Raising questions about antidepressants. *Psychother Psychosom.* **68**: 3–14.

5 Morgan SG, Bassett KL, Wright JM *et al.* (1005) 'Breakthrough' drugs and growth in expenditure on prescription drugs in Canada. *BMJ.* **331**: 815–6.

6 WHO Collaborating Centre for Drug Statistics Methodology (2004) *About the ATC/DDD system.* Last updated September 21, 2004. Available from www.whocc.no/atcddd (accessed November 8, 2005).

7 Patented Medicine Prices Review Board (2001) *Interprovincial Provincial Prescription Drug Price Comparison: 1995/96–1999/00.* PMPRB, Ottawa.

8 IMS Health Canada (2004) *Cholesterol Reducers again Fastest-Growing Class among Canada's Top Prescribed Drug Classes of 2003, 2004.* Available from www.imshealthcanada.com/htmen/3_1_40.htm (accessed March 15, 2004).

9 Oregon Health Resources Commission (2003) *HMG-CoA Reductase Inhibitors (STATINS) Report.* Update #1, September, 4.

10 Zhou Z, Rahme E, Abrahamowicz M *et al.* (2005) Effectiveness of statins for secondary prevention in elderly patients after acute myocardial infarction: an evaluation of class effect. *Can Med Assoc J.* **172**: 1195–6.

11 Schneeweiss S, Soumerai SB, Glynn RJ, Maclure M, Dormuth C and Walker AM (2002a) Impact of reference-based pricing for angiotensin-converting enzyme inhibitors on drug utilization. *Can Med Assoc J.* **166**: 737–45.

12 Schneeweiss S, Walker AM, Glynn RJ, Maclure M, Dormuth C and Soumerai SB (2002b) Outcomes of reference pricing for angiotensin-converting-enzyme inhibitors. *N Engl J Med.* **346**: 822–9.

13 IMS Health Canada (2004) *Healthpoints: hypertension.* Available from www.imshealthcanada.com/htmen/3_1_32.htm (accessed March 14, 2004).

14 TI (Therapeutics Initiative) newsletter #47 (2003) *The answer: thiazides first line for hypertension,* Jan-Mar. Available from www.ti.ubc.ca/pages/letter47.htm.

15 Law MR, Wald NJ, Morris JK and Jordan RE (2003) Value of low dose combination treatment with blood pressure lowering drugs: analysis of 354 randomised trials. *BMJ.* **326**: 1427.

16 Oregon Health Resources Commission (2003) *NSAIDs Subcommittee Report.* Update #1, August, 8. Available from www.oregonrx.org/OrgrxPDF/NSAIDS%20review/HRC%20Reports/NSAIDS%20Revision%201,%208–03.pdf (accessed March 14, 2004).

17 Smalley WE, Griffin MR, Fought RL, Sullivan L and Ray WA (1995) Effect of a prior-authorization requirement on the use of nonsteroidal antiinflammatory drugs by Medicaid patients. *N Engl J Med.* **332**: 1612–7.

18 Uhegarty K, Ames D, Anderson J, Johnson C, McKinnon R and Moulds R (2003) Use of antidepressant medications in the general practice setting. A critical review. *Aust Fam Physician.* **32**: 229–34, 236–7, 239.

19 Department of Health and Human Services (1999) US Public Health Services. *Mental Health: a Report of the Surgeon General. Specific Treatments for Episodes of Depression and Mania.* Chapter 4, section 3. Available from www.surgeongeneral.gov/library/mentalhealth/chapter4/sec3_2.html (accessed March 14, 2004).

20 Tamblyn RM, McLeod PJ, Abrahamowicz M, *et al.* (1994) Questionable prescribing for elderly patients in Quebec. *Can Med Assoc J.* **150**: 1801–9.

21 Denig P and Haaijer-Ruskamp FM (1995) Do physicians take cost into account when making prescribing decisions? *Pharmacoeconomics.* **8**: 282–90.

22 Safavi FT and Hayward RA (1992) Choosing between apples and apples: physicians' choices of prescription drugs that have similar side effects and efficacies. *J Gen Intern Med*. **7**: 32–7.

23 Lexchin J (1997) What information do physicians receive from pharmaceutical representatives? *Can Family Physician*. **43**: 941–5.

24 Prescrire International (2003) Performance of sales representatives in France: still bad. *Prescrire International*. **12**: 153–4.

25 Choudhry NK, Stelfox HT and Detsky AS (2002) Relationships between authors of clinical practice guidelines and the pharmaceutical industry. *JAMA*. **287**: 612–7.

26 Papanikolaou GN, Baltogianni MS, Contopoulos-Ioannidis DG, Haidich A-B, Giannakakis IA and Ioannidis JP (2001) Reporting of conflicts of interest in guidelines of preventive and therapeutic interventions. *BMC Med Res Methodol*. **1**: 3.

27 CBC TV (2002) *Targeting Doctors – Disclosure*. First broadcast, March 5.

28 Wolf H, Andreou P, Bata I *et al*. (1999) Trends in the prevalence and treatment of hypertension in Halifax County from 1985 to 1995. *Can Med Assoc J*. **161**: 699–704.

29 Wilson D (2005) New blood-pressure guidelines pay off – for drug companies. *Seattle Times*, June 26.

30 The ALLHAT Officers and Coordinators for the ALLHAT Collaborative Research Group (2002) Major outcomes in high-risk hypertensive patients randomized to angiotensin-converting enzyme inhibitor or calcium channel blocker vs diuretic: the antihypertensive and lipid-lowering treatment to prevent heart attack trial (ALLHAT). *JAMA*. **288**: 2981–97.

31 Tannenbaum H, Peloso P, Russell A and Marlow B (2000) An evidence-based approach to prescribing NSAIDs in the treatment of osteoarthritis and rheumatoid arthritis: The Second Canadian Consensus Conference. *Can J Clin Pharmacol*. **7** (Suppl. A): 4A–16A.

32 Ontario Drug Programs (2003) *2002/03 Report Card for the Ontario Drug Benefit Program*. Ontario Ministry of Health and Long-term Care, Toronto.

33 Patented Medicine Prices Review Board (2004) *PMPRB Annual Report 2003*. PMPRB, Ottawa.

34 Cassels A (2002) *Paying for What Works: BC's experience with the Reference Drug Program as a model for rational policy making*. Canadian Centre for Policy Alternatives, Vancouver, March.

35 Soumerai SB, Ross-Degnan D, Gortmaker S and Avorn J (1990) Withdrawing payment for nonscientific drug therapy. Intended and unexpected effects of a large-scale natural experiment. *JAMA*. **263**: 831–9.

36 Roughead EE, Gilbert AL and Primrose JG (1999) Improving drug use: a case study of events which led to changes in use of flucloxacillin in Australia. *Soc Sci Med*. **48**: 845–53.

37 Maclure M, Dormuth C, Naumann T *et al*. (1998) Influences of educational interventions and adverse news about calcium-channel blockers on first-line prescribing of antihypertensive drugs to elderly people in British Columbia. *Lancet*. **352**: 943–8.

38 May FW, Rowett DS, Gilbert AL, McNeece JI and Hurley E (1999) Outcomes of an educational-outreach service for community medical practitioners: non-steroidal anti-inflammatory drugs. *Med J Australia*. **170**: 471–4.

39 Oregon Health Resources Commission (2000) *Report on Strategies for Effective Management of Pharmaceuticals*. September 8. Available from www.ohppr.state.or.us/hrc/pdf/Misc.%20documents/ohrc_rpt.pdf (accessed March 14, 2004).

40 Morgan S (2005) Canadian prescription drug costs surpass 18 billion dollars. *Can Med Assoc J*. **172**: 1323–4.

Chapter 8

Statins: is the net being thrown too wide?

Andrew Thompson and Norman J. Temple

Introduction

It has been well known for several decades that a high blood level of cholesterol is a major risk factor for coronary heart disease (CHD). In most cases this can be corrected by diet. But why change your diet when you can achieve the same goal with a pill? Statins are highly effective at lowering the blood cholesterol level while also inducing other favorable changes in the blood lipid profile. For this reason they are heavily promoted for combating CHD.

These drugs are a modern success story. They are "the" medical treatment for CHD, both in prevention and therapy, and a superstar of the pharmaceutical industry with worldwide sales running at about $19 billion a year and growing. Truly, they are "blockbuster" drugs.

The effectiveness of statins: what do the clinical trials really tell us?

The huge financial success of statins not only profits the pharmaceutical industry but also all those whose finances and careers are furthered by the research and the sales. But to what extent is it also a success for the general public? To answer this we will look at the nine major long-term (five-year) clinical trials that have been carried out to establish the value of statins.[1–9] We will critically appraise the findings from these trials and attempt to decipher their meaning in terms of the cost-effectiveness of the use of statins for preventing CHD.

The comparison group: best current treatment or placebo control?

The control groups in all of the trials have been given placebo pills. However, for reasons explained in Chapter 2, where a therapy of proven value already exists, it should be given to the control group; placebos are not appropriate. For statins this "therapy" is not another drug but lifestyle factors. For example, the European Atherosclerosis Society 1987 guidelines argued that dietary management should be "the sole therapy for the majority of people with elevated levels [of blood lipids]."[10] A year later the US National Cholesterol Education Program[11] stated: "Drug therapy is likely to continue for many years, or for a lifetime. Hence, the decision to add drug therapy to the regimen should be made only after vigorous efforts at dietary treatment have not proven sufficient." Vigorous efforts are defined as "a minimum of six months of intensive dietary counseling" prior to initiating drug therapy.

These trials were initiated after the publication of these guidelines. But what the researchers did instead was to recommend dietary change, wait a few weeks – not six months – and then, if the blood cholesterol was still too high, enroll the subjects into the study proper. Efforts at dietary control of blood cholesterol fell far short of "vigorous."

The dietary guidelines were in effect during the time that these trials were carried out, yet they were not followed. Why? Was it only a matter of extra cost? Certainly, the initial cost would have been more, but from a patient-health perspective it would seem advisable to implement a dietary regime as this might not only help reduce CHD but could also have a beneficial impact on other diseases. The design of the studies suggests two possible errors in the results: first, if all the subjects had been given dietary intervention prior to commencing statins or placebos, it might have reduced the beneficial effect of statins; second, if the control group had been given diet therapy in addition to placebo, this might have narrowed the gap between it and the statin group.

The problem of endpoints

One of the most inconsistent aspects of the statin trials is the choice and variety of endpoints. These have been placed into more than a score of varying combinations with each other. For example, myocardial infarction (MI) and stroke are sometimes combined. Some studies include a treatment, usually a form of revascularization. Regrettably, there is no rigorous reporting of all-cause morbidity, nor of measurement of changes in overall quality of life in any of the studies. Instead, it is assumed that less CHD-related morbidity leads to less morbidity overall.

The most reliable and valuable measure is all-cause mortality; it is the one of primary concern to the recipients of the treatment – are they less likely to die soon, whatever the reason, if they take this drug? Unfortunately, it is not a commonly used measure. It is not even reported in a substudy of the Heart Protection Study and has to be searched for in several of the other trials.

Now there may well be good reasons why particular endpoints were chosen or not chosen. In particular, designing a trial that aims to demonstrate a significant reduction in all-cause mortality may be ideal from the perspective of providing clear results, but it requires a large sample sizes and this therefore much increases the cost of the trial. But the key point as far as this discussion is concerned is that the variety of endpoints does little to enhance the credibility of the results of these clinical trials.

Presenting the results

The way numbers are presented can make a major difference to how impressive the results appear. Let us consider one of the most successful trials in terms of reducing risk of CHD, namely the LIPID trial.[2] This trial involved only patients who already had CHD (i.e. it was a secondary prevention trial). The difference in deaths (from any cause) between the statin group and the placebo group was 3.1% over the course of six years. This is the absolute difference in risk and, for reasons explained in Chapter 2, is the most appropriate way to express results. But the impact of these results can be much magnified by expressing them as relative differences. In this trial 14.1% of the placebo group died and 11% in the statin drug group; this can be stated as: "The statin drug lowered the risk of death by 22%" (11 is 22% lower than 14.1). So a decrease of 3.1% has now become a rather dramatic 22% drop.

Another serious problem with the way the results are presented is that the reader is often not told the number needed to treat (NNT) for one patient to benefit. With the LIPID trial, for example, the absolute difference of 3.1% means the NNT is 32 (100/3.1). In other words, for a patient at this level of risk the odds that statins will prevent their death during the next six years are about one in 30. Presenting NNTs greatly facilitates making an informed judgment as to the true value of the medication.

With the 4S and LIPID trials the patients already had CHD and are therefore at high risk of dying from the disease. As a result the NNTs are fairly modest. Most such patients will probably therefore agree to take statins for years, even when given an unbiased version of the efficacy of the drug. But the situation is altogether different when we turn our attention to primary prevention trials. Here the subjects have one or more risk factors for CHD and are therefore at an elevated risk for the disease. However, their risk is still much lower than subjects in secondary prevention trials. It is at this point that the way that the benefits of statins are presented becomes of crucial importance. When the drop in risk of CHD with statins is expressed as relative risk, we find that it varies little with the type of patient: it falls by around 25% to 30% in both high-risk and low-risk patients. But this number tells us very little about how much real benefit an individual is likely to gain. As indicated in Table 8.1, the NNT for patients in the three primary prevention trials is much higher than is the case with secondary trials; in each case it is over 100. In actuality, the absolute difference in risk of CHD in primary prevention trials is really very small. In this situation the way the numbers are presented is likely to have a major impact on whether the patient agrees to take statins. Does the doctor say: "Mr Smith, if you take statins, this will reduce your risk of dying from heart disease by 30%"? Or does she say: "Mr Smith, if you take statins, then in seven years time there is a one chance in about 150 that your death will have been prevented"? We argue that the latter is a much more honest version of the clinical reality, but one that is far less likely to induce people to take the drug.

Another aspect of the way the results were calculated also requires comment. The subjects in these studies are, of course, free to quit at any time and this can profoundly affect the results. How should investigators handle that fact? The standard way to reduce investigator bias during a trial is to analyze the results according to "intention to treat" and look at the two groups as if everyone stayed true to their assigned treatment, drug or placebo. Not all investigators are happy with that.

This is most evident in the Heart Protection Study (HPS) where about one-third of the statin group quit taking statins during the trial and about one-third of the placebo group started taking statins.[5] The authors stated: "After making allowance for non-compliance, actual use of this regime [taking statins] would probably reduce these rates [of MI, stroke, and revascularization] by about one-third." This statement ignores possible differences between compliers and non-compliers. It assumes, in effect, that those who decided to quit taking their statin would have benefited just as much as those who complied. Similarly, it assumes that those in the placebo group who switched to taking a statin were as likely to benefit from the

Table 8.1 Statin drug trials

Trial	Type of trial	Patients	All-cause mortality*		CHD mortality*	
			Abs (%)	NNT	Abs (%)	NNT
4S[1]	Secondary		3.3	30	3.5	29
LIPID[2]	Secondary		3.1	32	1.9	53
CARE I[3]	Secondary		<1	>100	1.1	91
CARE II[4]	Secondary	Aged 65–75	Not reported		4.6	22
Heart Protection Study (HPS)[5]	Mainly secondary (14% primary; all diabetics)	35% with type 2 diabetes	1.8	56	1.5	67
Heart Protection Study (substudy)[6]	Mainly secondary (40% primary)	Type 2 diabetes	2.0	50	2.1	48†
WOSCOPS[7]	Primary		<1	>100	>1	>100
ALLHAT-LLT[8]	Primary	Hypertension	<1	>100	0.0	∞
AFCAPS/ TexCAPS[9]	Primary		<1	>100	<1	>100

CHD, coronary heart disease; Abs (%), absolute difference (in percent); NNT, number needed to treat.
* Data indicate differences between statin and placebo groups.
† All cardiovascular deaths (not just CHD).

statin as those already in the statin group. Such an interpretation assumes that any other difference between compliers and non-compliers is irrelevant. But there is no hard evidence for this. It is entirely possible that people's choices in taking or not taking statins may be associated with other factors that affect risk of CHD. For example, those who were assigned to the placebo group but then chose to take statins may have been people who tend to follow a relatively healthy lifestyle. If so, even if they had not taken statins, their risk of CHD would probably still have been low. If this is indeed the case, then the effect of this manipulation of the data is therefore to exaggerate the benefit of statins.

Cost-effectiveness of statins

Now let us look at the cost-effectiveness of statins for the prevention of CHD. A number of cost estimations have been made and these were recently reviewed by Luc Bonneux of Belgium, an author of a chapter in this book, and his colleagues.[12] The estimates vary by a wide margin based on several factors. A factor of major importance is the risk of the patient for CHD. The cost of statins for the prevention of CHD in high-risk patients was estimated as approximately $16 000 to $22 000 per year of life gained (based on 2001 prices). Such patients will typically already be in poor health, especially from prior CHD; we shall therefore assume that their quality of life is 0.8 (where 1 is perfect health). Based on this the cost per quality-adjusted years of life (QALY) is therefore around $22 000 to $30 000 (2005 prices). This makes statins an acceptable medical expense for such patients (based on our proposed cost limit, as stated in Chapter 1, of $50 000 per QALY as a medium-term goal, and $27 000 per QALY as both an ideal limit and a longer-term goal).

But a very different story emerges when we turn our attention to people at much lower risk of CHD. The above study[12] indicated that for patients at low or moderate risk of CHD, the cost per year of life gained is in the range $40 000 to $100 000. (As explained in the next section, when the investigators have been funded by the pharmaceutical industry, the cost estimates are usually suspiciously low and these have therefore been disregarded in favor of less biased estimates.) We shall assume that the quality of life of these patients is 0.85. This produces a cost per QALY of $51 000 to $128 000. This is several times higher than was the case with high-risk patients. The reason for this is simply a reflection of the much larger numbers for NNT in primary prevention trials (as compared to the high-risk subjects in secondary trials).

What these numbers demonstrate is that when patients at only modest risk of CHD are given statins, the drug can quickly become unacceptably expensive. This has become especially relevant because the latest National Cholesterol Education Program (NCEP) III guidelines (also known as ATP III guidelines) have widened the net for the use of statins.[13] According to a detailed analysis it was estimated that the new guidelines have the effect of expanding the number of people in the USA who are now eligible for lipid lowering by drug therapy (which in most cases means statins) from 15 million to 36 million.[14] For these extra 21 million people at only modest risk of CHD, the cost will be extremely high for the benefit achieved.

A major way in which the lower threshold was reached was by including smoking, hypertension, and diabetes as factors that help justify a prescription for statins. While these are indeed major risk factors for CHD, their inclusion may have been misguided. Each of these factors has its own set of treatment options, and these may not be fully exploited if people are now given statins. This was aptly pointed out by Abramson[15] in his response to the diabetes substudy of the HPS study:

> Still, there is a more fundamental difficulty with this study: What is its purpose? The study seems to be designed to provide value-free scientific evidence to guide doctors in the optimum care of their patients with diabetes, but there has been a sleight of hand. By focusing attention solely on the role of statins, doctors are distracted from far more beneficial and far less costly interventions.... The findings of multiple randomized studies have shown that ongoing diet and exercise counselling decrease the risk of developing type 2 diabetes by more than half.

Another intervention that is certainly many times more cost-effective than statins is aspirin. Marshall[16] noted that if patients at high risk of CHD are given aspirin, the cost of preventing a case of CHD by also giving statins becomes much higher. This is because as the risk of CHD of the patients has now been reduced by aspirin, the NNT for statins has increased, and the cost of statins to prevent CHD (as dollars per QALY) has therefore also much increased.

Based on these considerations the above cost estimations for use of statins may actually be *underestimations*. And adding to this suspicion is the problem with the research design of the clinical trials that we discussed earlier. If statins are, in fact, less effective for prevention of CHD than the clinical trials suggest, then the cost per QALY automatically increases.

Thus, a case can be made that statins are cost-effective for the small minority of people at especially high risk of CHD. However, the same cannot be said for throwing the net far and wide and including 36 million Americans (about one in six of all adults). This would certainly include people aged in their forties and fifties whose only risk factor is high cholesterol. Indeed, the drug companies are advertising on American TV directly to just that section of the population, urging them to ask their doctor for a prescription for statins. For people at that level of risk the cost of statins translates to well over $100 000 per QALY.

The most recent (2003) Canadian recommendations for treating high cholesterol levels also advocated what is, in effect, Rolls Royce medicine. An analysis of these recommendations shows that almost 600 000 Canadians at "low risk" and a similar number at "moderate risk" are now eligible for statin therapy; the NNTs to prevent one CHD-related death in five years are 1550 and 366, respectively.[17]

Conflict of interest and guidelines on the use of statins

It is noteworthy that many of the people involved in writing guidelines that recommend large increases in the numbers of people given statin therapy also have links with pharmaceutical companies that make these drugs. The Chair of the committee that wrote the NCEP[13] guidelines, as well as five of the 13 members of the committee, has received drug-company funding. Similarly, the *BMJ* reported: "Guidelines for lowering cholesterol concentrations, issued [in 2004] by the National Heart, Lung, and Blood Institute and the American Heart Association, sparked a furore when it was shown that all but one of the nine authors had financial ties to the manufacturers of cholesterol lowering drugs."[18] This indicates that conflict of interest may be a significant factor in the writing of guidelines that have turned statins into a goldmine for the pharmaceutical industry.

Conflict of interest also seems to have been a major factor when it comes to making estimates of the cost-effectiveness of statins for the prevention of CHD. Making these calculations involves so many variables and assumptions that it is quite easy to double or halve the bottom line. We referred above to a review paper by Luc Bonneux and colleagues[12] that looked at the various analyses that have been made. One of their findings was that for people at low-to-moderate risk of CHD, the source of funding of the study was a major factor in determining the stated cost-effectiveness of statins. They found that when the investigators who published the estimates were funded by government or universities, the cost of statins, relative to benefit achieved, was around two to four times higher than when the funding came from the pharmaceutical industry. This strongly suggests that the drug manufacturers have exerted undue influence so that published estimates make statins appear to be much better value for money than they really are.

Conclusions

The trials testing statins have not followed the guideline-recommended promotion of lifestyle changes before instituting the drugs. The differences favoring statins have been magnified by the manner of presentation of results, namely the use of relative risk differences between statins and placebo groups rather than absolute differences. Lowering the threshold to make much larger numbers of people eligible for drug therapy has the effect of making the use of statins extremely expensive to achieve the prevention of CHD. This seems less of a benefit than a misguided approach that is potentially wasteful of billions of dollars. The case for statins, certainly for primary prevention where the risk of death from CHD is not especially high, has not been made.

For patients at relatively high risk of CHD aspirin is far more cost-effective than statins. Aspirin appears to lower the risk of CHD, especially in men.[19] In women it appears to mainly reduce the risk of stroke.[19] So why, we may ask, is there more aggressive promotion of statins rather than aspirin? The obvious explanation is because of the difference in profit margins.

References

1 Scandinavian Simvastatin Survival Study Group (1994) Randomized trial of cholesterol lowering in 4444 patients with coronary heart disease: the Scandinavian Simvastatin Survival Study. *Lancet.* **344**: 1383–9.

2 The Long-Term Intervention with Pravastatin in Ischemic Disease (LIPID) Study Group (1998) Prevention of cardiovascular events and death with pravastatin in patients with coronary heart disease and a broad range of initial cholesterol levels. *N Engl J Med.* **339**: 1349–57.

3 Sacks FM, Pfeffer MA, Moye LA *et al.* (1996) The effect of pravastatin on coronary events after myocardial infarction in patients with average cholesterol levels. *N Engl J Med.* **335**: 1001–9.

4 Lewis SJ, Moye LA, Sacks FM *et al.* (1998) Effect of pravastatin on cardiovascular events in older patients with myocardial infarction and cholesterol levels in the average range. Results of the Cholesterol and Recurrent Events (CARE) trial. *Ann Intern Med.* **129**: 681–9.

5 Heart Protection Study Collaborative Group (2002) MRC/BHF Heart Protection Study of cholesterol lowering with simvastatin in 20,536 high-risk individuals: a randomized placebo-controlled trial. *Lancet.* **360**: 7–22.

6 Collins R, Armitage J, Parish S *et al.* (2003) MRC/BHF Heart Protection Study of cholesterol-lowering with simvastatin in 5963 people with diabetes: a randomised placebo-controlled trial. *Lancet.* **361**: 2005–16.

7 Shepherd, J, Cobbe SM, Ford I *et al.* (1995) Prevention of coronary heart disease with pravastatin in men with hypercholesterolemia. *N Engl J Med.* **333**: 1301–7.

8 ALLHAT Officers and Coordinators for the ALLHAT Collaborative Research Group (2002) Major outcomes in moderately hypercholesterolemic, hypertensive patients randomized to pravastatin vs usual care: the Antihypertensive and Lipid-Lowering Treatment to Prevent Heart Attack Trial (ALLHAT-LLT). *JAMA.* **288**: 2998–3007.

9 Downs JR, Clearfield M, Weis S *et al.* (1998) Primary prevention of acute coronary events with lovastatin in men and women with average cholesterol levels: results of AFCAPS/TexCAPS. Air Force/Texas Coronary Atherosclerosis Prevention Study. *JAMA.* **279**: 1615–22.

10 European Atherosclerosis Society (1987) Strategies for the prevention of coronary heart disease: a policy statement of the European Atherosclerosis Society. *Eur Heart J.* **8**: 77–88.

11 Expert Panel (1988) Report of the National Education Program Expert Panel on detection, evaluation, and treatment of high blood cholesterol in adults. The Expert Panel. *Arch Intern Med.* **148**: 36–69.

12 Franco OH, Peeters A, Looman CW and Bonneux L (2005) Cost effectiveness of statins in coronary heart disease. *J Epidemiol Community Health.* **59**: 927–33.

13 National Cholesterol Education Program (NCEP) (2002) Third Report of the National Cholesterol Education Program (NCEP) Expert Panel on Detection, Evaluation, and Treatment of High Blood Cholesterol in Adults (Adult Treatment Panel III) final report. *Circulation.* **106**: 3143–421.

14 Fedder DO, Koro CE and L'Italien GJ (2002) New National Cholesterol Education Program III guidelines for primary prevention lipid-lowering drug therapy: projected impact on the size, sex, and age distribution of the treatment-eligible population. *Circulation.* **105**: 152–6.
15 Abramson J (2003) Comments on the MRC/BHF Heart Protection Study. *Lancet.* **362**: 745–6.
16 Marshall T (2003) Coronary heart disease prevention: insights from modelling incremental cost effectiveness. *BMJ.* **327**: 1264.
17 Manuel DG, Tanuseputro P, Mustard CA *et al.* (2005) The 2003 Canadian recommendations for dyslipidemia management: revisions are needed. *Can Med Assoc J.* **172**: 1027–31.
18 Lenzer J (2004) Scandals have eroded US public's confidence in drug industry. *BMJ.* **329**: 247.
19 Ridker PM, Cook NR, Lee IM *et al.* (2005) A randomized trial of low-dose aspirin in the primary prevention of cardiovascular disease in women. *N Engl J Med.* **352**: 1293–304.

Chapter 9

Modern Western medicine: lots of bucks – where's the bang?

Norman J. Temple and Joy Fraser

Introduction

Modern medicine has indisputably delivered huge benefits. Few of us would hesitate before seeking medical assistance for a condition such as cancer or a serious injury. During the last half-century an enormous number of medical innovations have contributed clinically and economically to developed nations, and with the use of modern technologies we have conquered or diminished the effects of many horrible and incurable diseases. There is no question that improved diagnostic techniques and new treatments, including new drugs, have enabled millions of people to live longer and enjoy a better quality of life. Through all of these developments medicine has tried its utmost, and with much success, to place itself atop the podium of public esteem. But that does not mean that medicine should escape critical evaluation.

In this chapter we examine some of the problem areas in medicine, such as the drug industry, physicians, and also some of the wider medical structures of which physicians are the front line. While our main focus is cost-effectiveness, we also look at other aspects, such as safety and efficacy.

As university professors, at least in our university, we must carefully monitor the cost of everything we want to do. If we choose a particular textbook for a course, then we must state its cost as part of the plan we present to a larger university community for course development approval. And the same applies in many other areas. Teachers, for example, are seldom allowed to forget that their schools operate on a tight budget and they must plan their school year accordingly. But medicine often seems to operate by a different rulebook, one in which cost is simply not a relevant issue. Alas, physicians, both in North America and more globally, are not much better than the US military, which has been notorious for buying its war toys with what seems to be total disregard for cost. In medicine, there are many ways that money is spent carelessly, but the relationship with drugs is clearly the most blatant manifestation of this problem and the most insidious.

Drugs

"Pharmaceutical companies will soon rule the world if we keep letting them believe we are a happy, functional society so long as all the women are on Prozac, all children on Ritalin, and all men on Viagra."[1]

Drugs: how big is the problem?

In several of the previous chapters we have documented the extent to which the entire pharmaceutical system – from research, through drug approval by regulatory agencies, to marketing, and, finally, to the prescribing habits of physicians – leads to a colossal waste of money. And it is not hard to see why. As we follow the path that new drugs take as they progress from the laboratory to being prescribed as a treatment, we see abundant evidence of a system in need of radical reform. In a nutshell, when the research evidence concerning the value of a particular drug is distorted, drugs of inferior value (or even dangerous) compared to alternative but cheaper drugs, can be hyped as superior. And that, of course, inevitably means that real folks pay the price – not only in highly inflated costs when purchasing drugs but the price in terms of adverse side effects and even death. Unfortunately, we have a serious lack of hard numbers and this prevents us from quantifying the rate at which money is being flushed down the drain, or, more accurately, into the hugely inflated profit margins of the pharmaceutical companies.

The statistics on drugs are astounding. Wolfe[2] estimated that 3.4 billion prescriptions were filled in drugstores and by mail order in the USA in 2003, averaging out to 11.7 prescriptions filled for every one of the 290 million people who live there. But we know that many people did not fill any prescriptions that year, which means that others had an overabundance of prescriptions – and these were mainly the elderly. Stagnitti[3] found that the elderly used more than twice as many drugs (23.5 prescriptions per year) as those aged under 65 years. Overall, half of all Americans take at least one prescription medicine on any given day, while 27% take three or more.[4]

In a report on healthcare expenses for the Agency for Healthcare Research and Quality in the USA, Ezzati-Rice *et al.*[5] reported that, in the year 2000, civilian, noninstitutionalized Americans spent approximately $103 billion on 2.2 billion prescriptions. The people who used prescription drugs spent an average of $594 each that year. When drug use in hospitals and nursing homes is included, the actual cost of drugs in the USA is substantially higher.

Who is to blame?

In order to properly comprehend the problem, we need to look at the entire system, from drug development, at one end, to the issuing of prescriptions to patients, at the other. What is the mindset of the actors at each stage? We can divide the key players into the following groups, which together have created a near-perfect storm.

Scientists conducting basic research and drug trials

Although these are the folks who get the ball rolling, they are perhaps the least responsible for the problems that develop "downstream." Their motivation is, in the great majority of cases, honest and sincere. By the very nature of research that may lead to a new drug, or in the testing of a newly developed drug, it is very hard to predict how things will eventually turn out. And, except in cases where special factors make it predictable that the cost of a new drug is going to be extremely high, it is especially difficult for researchers to foresee the cost-effectiveness of new treatments. But it does happen that researchers engaged in clinical trials do participate in unethical behavior in the service of the pharmaceutical industry. There are several ways by which this can be done, and which were discussed in chapters 2 and 3; for example, enrolling certain types of patients for a trial in order to improve the odds of generating the "right" results, not publishing results that reveal problems with the new drug, or allowing data to be published that somehow exaggerate the benefits of the drug. The researchers who engage in such actions are typically motivated by either financial rewards or by career enhancement.

Movers and shakers in the pharmaceutical industry

The evidence from previous chapters makes it quite apparent that these are the people largely responsible for the grossly excessive costs and huge waste inherent in so much drug treatment. They engineer the entire system so that their "me-too" drugs are quickly put through clinical trials, medical journals publish the results that fail to tell the whole story, drugs are approved for uses where the supporting evidence is dubious, and marketing is done so as to maximize sales of those drugs that generate high profits. For these people, the cost-effectiveness of the therapy is more of an obstacle than a goal.

Those between the pharmaceutical industry and the front-line physicians

These are the experts on drug therapy who write review papers and formulate guidelines, the journal editors who decide what will be published, and the government officials who decide which drugs will be approved. The pharmaceutical companies have developed great expertise in manipulating these groups. In the words of Napoleon: "Every man has his price." When you have a huge budget for marketing drugs, there are many ways to ensure that the desired message is delivered to the right audience. By such tactics as funding medical researchers to conduct clinical trials to "prove" the efficacy of particular drugs, making payments to experts so that these drugs get favorable reviews in medical journals and are recommended in clinical practice guidelines, and by making journals dependent on advertising revenue, overpriced drugs of questionable value and unproven safety can be made to look like therapeutic advances.

Physicians

Those trying to decide which drugs to prescribe have a tough job. They are constantly fed large volumes of carefully crafted marketing material, often conveying the message that newer and more expensive drugs are better, with the primary aim of persuading them to write prescriptions. In the USA physicians must contend with patients who request drugs after seeing them advertised on television. Added to this, physicians usually lack the time to make fully informed choices. It is hardly surprising, therefore, that their prescribing habits end up causing a great deal of money to be squandered. Nevertheless, as we shall see, physicians are far from blameless in their prescribing habits.

Physicians are the gatekeepers of the entire medical system, and it is they who must bear much of the blame for the serious problems discussed here. The problem starts in medical school and continues through the everyday work of physicians; seldom is any emphasis given to issues of cost-effectiveness. What should be done about this sorry state of affairs? Later chapters propose some answers to this question. One essential component of the solution will be the injection of appropriate additions to the curriculum at medical schools.

One of the fundamental problems that is often overlooked is the failure of medical practitioners and governments to recognize and embrace health promotion and illness prevention strategies; instead, there is a profound bias toward prescribing drugs and other medical interventions. In place of health promotion we have drug promotion!

A closer look at drug problems

The problem of enormous financial waste has been the dominant theme in several previous chapters. But the misuse of drug therapy extends well beyond problems of overspending. The overuse of drugs is a dangerous trend, contributing to some of our most serious health problems.

The elderly are the group most likely to be the victims of inappropriate prescribing, often as a result of an adverse drug reaction being misinterpreted as a new medical condition and then a new drug being prescribed. This domino effect is referred to as the "prescribing cascade"[6] and results in serious adverse effects and drug-induced diseases, such as Parkinsonism, depression, insomnia, and psychoses. Besides the health risks, it also results in an enormous amount of financial waste.

A serious problem pertains to the huge overprescribing of antibiotics. While this problem may have moderated somewhat in recent years, over- and inappropriate prescribing practices are still pervasive. In a study of patients visiting community-based outpatient clinics the researchers concluded that: "Antibiotic use in ambulatory patients is decreasing in the United States. However, physicians are increasingly turning to expensive, broad-spectrum agents, even when there is little clinical rationale for their use."[7] Nyquist et al.[8] studied a representative sample of ambulatory care physicians in the USA and confirmed that despite recommendations to the contrary, there was widespread overprescribing of antibiotics for children with colds, upper respiratory infections, and bronchitis. Schwartz et al.[9] pointed to research which showed that the overuse of antibiotics results in increased costs, adverse drug reactions, and treatment failures in patients with antibiotic-resistant infections. They suggested that educational programs for both physicians and parents might help remedy this problem if carried out in conjunction with specific policies that promote more judicious use of antibiotics, such as using appropriate tests to diagnose Group A streptococcal infections before prescribing drugs. However, in an analysis of American children with a sore throat between 1997 and 2003, Linder et al.[10] found no association between the performance of a recommended test for Group A -hemolytic streptococci (GABHS) and antibiotic prescribing. Physicians prescribed antibiotics to 53% of the children they saw, of which 27% were non-recommended antibiotics. These authors concluded that the overall prescribing rates continue to exceed the expected prevalence of GABHS, and broad-spectrum antibiotics were selected unnecessarily despite access to an objective test to guide the treatment of children with sore throats.

We know that the continued misuse of antibiotics not only results in increased costs and waste, but, more importantly, the use of unnecessary antibiotics exposes patients to adverse drug events and increases the prevalence of antibiotic-resistant bacteria. Moreover, Howard and Scott[11] suggest that to date we cannot even measure the complete burden to society of drug resistance due to inappropriate antibiotic use.

Pressure from parents is a major reason for unnecessary and inappropriate prescribing practices for children. However, other factors, such as concerns about malpractice lawsuits and dealing with busy schedules, also contribute to their unwise decisions to prescribe antibiotics for infections when there is no evidence that they will be effective.

Medicine: too much of a moderately good thing?

Used sensibly, medicine is of tremendous value and can prevent many deaths. Alas, there is strong evidence that a large part of the American population suffers from a gross excess of supply and, consequently, there is an enormous amount of needless and wasted expenditure. Strong supporting evidence for this comes from studies done by Fisher and colleagues.[12,13] These investigators studied the relationship between medical expenditures and outcomes for almost a million patients spread across the USA who suffered from one of three conditions, namely, acute myocardial infarction, hip fracture, or colorectal cancer. There were major variations in the cost of treatment and this was accounted for mainly by the number of consultations, tests, and hospitalization days. An analysis of the data revealed that patients in high-cost areas fared no better with respect to five-year mortality rates, functional status, or quality of care. Indeed, if anything, areas with higher medical expenditures tended to have higher mortality rates. The findings indicate that if every health area reduced its costs to the level of the areas with the lowest costs, as much as 30% of healthcare costs might be saved. And that is without considering massive overcharging on drugs. This astonishing finding is of profound importance. Of course, further research is required to verify specific factors. But this study provides strong evidence that huge amounts of medical interventions are carried out, not because they are actually required based on proven need, but rather because the supply is there and physicians then go ahead and utilize it.

Alan Sager and Deborah Socolar,[14] two researchers from Boston University School of Public Health, took a broader look at wasteful overspending by the American medical system. They considered all aspects of this, including administrative costs and overcharging. They concluded that about half of healthcare spending is eaten up by waste, excessive prices, and fraud. In addition to huge amounts of wasteful spending, there are costs related to poor medical practices and enhanced patient risk within the healthcare system.

The boast is often heard that "America has the best medical system in the world." The hollowness of this statement was exposed by an analysis published in *JAMA* in 2000 by Barbara Starfield.[15] She estimated that 225 000 people die in the USA each year from iatrogenic causes, mostly from infections contracted in hospitals, and from adverse effects of medications (actual errors in giving medication were disregarded). Incredible as it may seem, this makes iatrogenic causes the third leading cause of death in the USA, well ahead of stroke. This finding should rate a 9.2 on the Richter scale. It speaks volumes as to the arrogance inherent in so much of the American medical system. Another informative study concluded that the annual cost of drug-related morbidity and mortality in the USA was $177 billion in 2000.[16]

And Canada is not much better. A large Canadian study suggests that healthcare can be hazardous to our health judging by the rates of adverse events (AE) among hospitalized patients. Baker and colleagues[17] randomly selected four acute care hospitals of different sizes in each of five provinces and reviewed a random selection of charts for AE. These were defined as an "unintended injury or complication that results in disability at the time of discharge, death, and/or prolonged hospital stay, and that is caused by healthcare management rather than by the patient's underlying disease process." According to their findings, nearly 70 000 admissions annually in Canada are associated with a preventable adverse event. The most common types were related to surgical procedures, followed by drug- or fluid-related events. Most patients who experienced AE had longer hospital stays or suffered temporary disabilities; however, over 5% of the AE resulted in permanent disability and 16% resulted in death. These results led the researchers to estimate that in similar hospitalizations in Canada, death would be associated with an adverse event in 1.6% of patients. Davis[18] points out that the high incidence of AE exposes the paradox that currently exists in healthcare: by lavishing more healthcare on patients, we are not only incurring huge costs, we are placing people at great risk.

Medicine: a system in need of repair

Bannerman et al.[19] remind us that the USA is the wealthiest nation on earth. Its per capita spending on healthcare is more than that of any other country. Yet, despite this, it is the only country in the industrialized world where its people do not have access to a universal healthcare system and, as a result, they live in fear of a disastrous event that could leave them destitute. Even those with jobs and good health plans run into problems since coverage has been cut back by health maintenance organizations and insurance companies, while costs for drugs, diagnostic services, hospitals, and health providers have soared. These huge amounts spent on healthcare do not add up to high quality of care. The USA is rated below other countries when it comes to the health of its citizens, especially in its treatment of the poor and its ethnic minority groups. One of the most revealing statistics upon which the health of a nation is gauged is the infant mortality rate. The overall infant mortality rate in the USA is 6.7 deaths per 1000 – a ranking of 24th in the world. But among American blacks it is 14 per 1000, making it the 77th in the world, as low as Belarus and Bulgaria.[19] (Canada is ranked at 15 with 5 deaths per 1000.)

Research!America[20] found high levels of dissatisfaction with the healthcare system. In their national 2005 survey, 60% of Americans said they no longer believe that the USA has the best healthcare system in the world and 64% said that people do not get the health and medical care they need. Woolley and Propst[21] noted that in a CBS/New York Times poll[22] healthcare overall was rated one of the most important domestic issues (28%), with education (22%) and jobs (20%) following behind. However, the cost of healthcare was identified as the leading concern. This is consistent with findings from a survey conducted jointly by USA Today, the Kaiser Family Foundation, and Harvard School of Public Health. This found that large numbers of Americans have serious worries about healthcare costs.[4] For example,

28% of adults were unable to pay for some form of medical care in the past year, a proportion that has almost doubled since 1976.

Access to healthcare is viewed as a basic human right, but it is steadily becoming more expensive than the average person can afford. The poor and the elderly are especially affected by high healthcare costs and have reduced access to quality care, including medications, compared to the more affluent.

References

1   Guillemets T (2005) *Quote Garden.* Available from www.quotegarden.com/drugs.html (accessed November 10, 2005).
2   Wolfe S (2005) Misprescribing and Overprescribing of Drugs. Public Citizen's Health Research Group. Available from www.worstpills.org/public/page.cfm?op_id=3# (accessed November 11, 2005).
3   Stagnitti MN (2004) *Trends in Outpatient Prescription Drug Utilization and Expenditures: 1997–2000.* Statistical Brief #21, February 2004. Agency for Healthcare Research and Quality, Rockville, MD. Available from www.meps.ahrq.gov/PrintProducts/PrintProdLookup.asp?ProductType=StatisticalBrief (accessed November 11, 2005).
4   Kaiser Family Foundation (2005) *Health Care Costs Survey, 2005.* Available from www.kff.org/newsmedia/pomr090105pkg.cfm (accessed November 15, 2005).
5   Ezzati-Rice TM, Kashihara D and Machlin SR (2004) *Expenses in the United States, 2000.* Research Findings #21: Health Care, April. Agency for Healthcare Research and Quality, Rockville, MD. Available from www.meps.ahrq.gov/papers/rf21_04–0022/rf21.htm (accessed November 11, 2005).
6   Rochon PA and Gurwitz JH (1997) Optimizing drug treatment for elderly people: the prescribing cascade. *BMJ.* **315:** 1096–9.
7   Steinman MA, Gonzales R, Linder JA and Landefeld CS (2003) Changing use of antibiotics in community-based outpatient practice, 1991–1999. *Ann Intern Med.* **138:** 525–33.
8   Nyquist AC, Gonzales R, Steiner JF *et al.* (1998) Antibiotic prescribing for children with colds, upper respiratory tract infections, and bronchitis. *JAMA.* **279:** 875–7.
9   Schwartz B, Mainous AG and Marcy SM (1998) Why do physicians prescribe antibiotics for children with upper respiratory tract infections? *JAMA.* **279:** 881–2.
10 Linder JA, Bates DW, Lee GM *et al.* (2005) Antibiotic treatment of children with sore throat. *JAMA.* **294:** 2315–22.
11 Howard DH and Scott DR (2005) The economic burden of drug resistance. *Clin Infect Dis.* **41**(Suppl. 4): S283–6.
12 Fisher ES, Wennberg DE, Stukel TA *et al.* (2003a) The implications of regional variations in Medicare spending. Part 1: the content, quality, and accessibility of care. *Ann Intern Med.* **138:** 273–87.
13 Fisher ES, Wennberg DE, Stukel TA *et al.* (2003b) The implications of regional variations in Medicare spending. Part 2: health outcomes and satisfaction with care. *Ann Intern Med.* **138:** 288–98.
14 Sagar A and Socolar D (2005) *Health Costs Absorb One-quarter of Economic Growth, 2000–2005.* Health Reform Program, School of Public Health, Boston University, Boston, MA. Available from http://dcc2.bumc.bu.edu/hs/ushealthreform.htm (accessed November 6, 2005).
15 Starfield B (2000) Is US health really the best in the world? *JAMA.* **284:** 483–5.
16 Ernst FR and Grizzle AJ. (2001) Drug-related morbidity and mortality: updating the cost-of-illness model. *J Am Pharm Assoc.* **41:** 192–9.
17 Baker GR, Norton PG, Flintoft V *et al.* (2004) The Canadian Adverse Events Study: the incidence of adverse events among hospital patients in Canada. *Can Med Assoc J.* **170:** 1678–86.
18 Davis P (2004) Health care as a risk factor. *Can Med Assoc J.* **170:** 1688–9.
19 Bannerman G, Nixdorf DC and Waghorn K (2005) *Squandering Billions: health care in Canada.* Hancock House Publishers, Surrey, BC.
20 Research!America (2005) *Health Poll. Taking Our Pulse: the PARADE,* June. Available from http://archive.parade.com/2005/0710/0710_index.html (accessed November 11, 2005).

21 Woolley M and Propst SM (2005) Public attitudes and perceptions about health-related research. *JAMA*. **294**: 1380–4.

22 CBS News/*New York Times* (2005) Poll, June 10–15. Available from www.pollingreport.com/prioriti.htm (accessed November 11, 2005).

Note by the editors

The large majority of the contents of chapters 3–9 has dealt with problems related to the pharmaceutical industry and the drugs it markets. Chapter 9 began a change of focus, namely to other problem areas where the way in which medicine conducts its business leads to various problems, especially with regard to excessive and wasteful spending. This discussion continues in the next several chapters.

The focus of Chapter 10 is the brave new world of genomic medicine. This includes two major areas: genetic testing that attempts to identify individuals who have genes that make them susceptible to particular diseases; gene therapy where researchers seek new wonder cures that will fix the problem.

In chapters 11–14 we turn our attention to screening for cancer. This is another area that makes grand promises, notably a sizeable reduction in deaths from cancer, but costs billions while also being far from risk-free. Whereas genomic medicine is still at the drawing board stage, screening for cancer is very much here and now. As with other topics, such as the use of statins, we will attempt to answer the questions:

How effective is screening for cancer for improving health and reducing the risk of major disease?

To what extent is the cost justified for the benefit delivered?

Chapter 10

Genetics, genomic medicine, and achieving better population health: a flawed strategy

Patricia A. Baird and Norman J. Temple

Please note that the following is a short version of this chapter, the full version can be found on the Radcliffe website (www.radcliffe-oxford.com/medicalspending).

Genetic testing: summary and recommendations

Of course, the goal of preventing the diseases that make up most of the population disease burden is a worthy one. However, a genetic approach is seriously limited in what it can achieve.[1,2] For the foreseeable future, widespread genetic susceptibility testing would not be an ethical or appropriate use of resources – it would provide minimal benefit at too high a cost and has the potential to cause much harm. A much better use of limited resources is to focus on supporting people in living healthier lives and improving the environment for everyone. This is explored in Chapter 16.

Despite the lack of solid evidence in support of population-based genetic testing there is growing pressure to market this technology. Many of the claims for such genetic screening tests are made by parties who stand to gain: laboratories, service providers, biotechnology firms, and scientists working in genetics. Companies interested in predictive diagnostic DNA tests are likely to be the ones who are also developing drug interventions to prevent or treat the disease to be predicted. There is potentially a huge market for predictive diagnostic DNA tests done on a large proportion of the healthy population to assess their "risk" status. Simplistic perceptions that "genes cause disease" lead to a population of consumers ripe for marketing of gene-based diagnostics and products. The public needs to be street-proofed.

As yet, no legislation prevents a company from marketing what it claims to be predictive genetic tests for hundreds of different diseases. If genetic testing is not simply just another market commodity, regulation is needed. At the present stage of development there is a chance to anticipate and shape the area of genetic "susceptibility" testing by regulations and clear policies. Guidelines and safeguards should be established to ensure that if such testing takes place, it will be done in an ethical and beneficial manner[3] with fully informed consent, and that testing will not be driven solely by commercial goals. There should also be legal protections against workplace and insurance discrimination. There is a risk that some employers may perceive genetic testing as a way to reduce their costs by decreasing the number of sick employees or compensation claims. Other regulatory actions are needed with regard to direct-to-consumer advertising, which should be limited and should meet predetermined standards and guidelines.

Genomic medicine: concluding comments

We are at an exciting time in genetics. There have been remarkable advances in our knowledge and there will certainly be real benefits from a carefully considered application of genetic knowledge in the future. Steady progress in unraveling the mysteries locked in our DNA will allow us, in some specific instances, to ameliorate particular disease processes or use medication more effectively. However, policy makers should view new and expanded expenditures in the area of genetic testing and therapy with the question of cost in mind, a healthy scepticism, and an evaluation of who is advocating such expenditures and whether they are ones who will gain. Genetics is only part of the story, and it is important to evaluate genetic components to disease causation within a wider context.

There is a serious problem with conflict of interest in all areas of genomic medicine, both genetic testing and gene therapy, as large commercial enterprises are involved that have a vested interest in pushing their own agenda regardless of the greater good. As long as companies can turn a short-term profit, testing, gadgetry, products, and procedures will be marketed, and marketed aggressively, almost regardless of worth. Unless appropriate regulation and monitoring is put in place, they will only be withdrawn if they are shown to lead to near-future, provable harm. In the meantime, it is important to support research into the dietary, behavioral, socioeconomic, and environmental factors that strongly affect the frequency of most common diseases. Such research is likely to continue to generate many advances that reveal how these diseases can be prevented, and in many cases treated. The hard truth is that, for the great majority of us, far more is likely to be achieved by gym therapy than by gene therapy.

References

1 Beaglehole R (2001) Global cardiovascular disease prevention: time to get serious. *Lancet.* **358**: 661–3.
2 Baird PA (2001) Current challenges to appropriate clinical use of new genetic knowledge in different countries. *Community Genet.* 4: 12–7.
3 Zimmern R, Emery J and Richards T (2001) Putting genetics in perspective. *BMJ.* **322**: 1005–6.

Chapter 11

Issues in screening for cancer

Luc Bonneux

Introduction

Health economics is a young science. Economics is actually a social science which implies that the evidence base is more "soft" than the empirical data of clinical epidemiology. This opens the door for abuse by industry or interest groups, which manipulate data and models for advancing their own aims. This chapter will demonstrate that the assumptions of linearity underlying cancer models fit the a priori assumption that cancer screening is useful. In the cancer models used in economic evaluation, the central assumption is changed to the main result. I am not aware of evaluation models based on true, evolutionary models of carcinogenesis (chaotic mutations and nonrandom selection for aggressiveness);[1,2] it would be easy to define such a model with the a priori hypothesis that cancer screening is not useful. Of course, neither approach has much to do with unbiased scientific evaluation.

Challenges in assessing cancer screening

In economic analysis of the cost of health effects, there are two main methods: "primary" and "secondary" analysis.[3] In primary analysis, costs and effects are directly obtained from observations (e.g. a randomized clinical trial, RCT). These findings give reliable estimates of the reality observed in a RCT, with tenuous external validity in the real world of average doctors, general hospitals, and so forth. Primary analysis measures costs and effects of both arms of a RCT. It reveals whether or not, at least in the conditions of a RCT, a treatment is cost-effective. Such analysis is less open to bias and is the most reliable. However, primary analysis is impossible in cancer screening. Any primary analysis would highlight a very interesting problem: that the potential "signals" of event changes by cancer screening are drowned in the noise of concurrent morbidity and competing mortality. Failure to recognize that problem besets all cancer screening research. Even in the best case of good effectiveness, an absolute mortality risk reduction in a frequent single cancer type is still a small effect in a large pool of degenerative disorders rapidly emerging in middle-aged and elderly populations. In a country with high breast cancer mortality, the probability of dying of breast cancer in a low-risk population of women, eligible in case of population-wide screening, is about 2%.[4] Note that this excludes women younger than 50 (generally not included in population-based screening programs as there is no evidence of effectiveness) and women who are at high risk because of familial or other disorders. Population-based screening typically addresses women that have no increased risk of breast cancer and hence no clinical reason for medical surveillance. A reduction of 25% will therefore reduce all-cause mortality by 0.5%. It is impossible to prove such small changes beyond a reasonable doubt.[5] Cancer epidemiologists wishing to debate the results of cancer screening may look forward to an infinite future of "yes," "no," and "maybe" papers.

In secondary analysis, costs and effects are generated by a simulation model. The principle is that any model will construct and compare synthetic cohorts with and without screening. Tumor history is unknown so an imagined linear model is constructed: small tumors do not metastastize and kill; small tumors become big tumors; big tumors metastasize and kill.[6] It is evident that in such a model screening is highly effective.[7] Any discovered tumor is a prevented cancer death. The problem with this is that carcinogenesis is not a linear process but an evolutionary one.[1] Random damage promotes uninhibited cell growth, which is continuously emerging and eliminated by cellular defence mechanisms. Aggressive cancer is selected for by inefficient elimination. One of the implications is that the sooner you intervene in the carcinogenic process, the less likely it is that cell lines will grow into an aggressive cancer. However, while early diagnosis and intervention will lead to (superfluous) treatment of benign disease, it will not necessarily lead to successful treatment of malignant disease. Any tumor that can be discovered by macroscopic imaging contains billions of cells and represents a cell line that has existed for years.[8] If it has acquired the potential for aggressive metastasis, then metastasis may already have occurred and treatment of the primary tumor will then be too little, too late.

Secondary analysis is a cost hypothesis "analysis:" an analysis of a hypothetical set of assumptions. Such models, used inductively, are unscientific as they cannot be falsified: they are built on contentious assumptions. Different assumptions will lead to other results. But there is no way to decide which model is good or which is bad. The US Preventive Services Task Force recently reviewed the cost-effectiveness of breast cancer screening in women over 65 year of age: they found more than 60 studies, 10 that were "acceptable" and that showed more than 10-fold differences in cost-effectiveness ratios.[9]

Fundamental principles of cancer screening

To understand cancer screening it is necessary to understand the underlying dynamics in terms of distributions of growth and metastasis rates. Carcinogenesis creates more or less aggressive cell lines, with slow or rapid tumor growth, inclined or disinclined to metastasis, and vulnerable or not vulnerable to the defensive attacks of the organism. But none of these parameters can be predicted. If a tumor is detected as a consequence of a complaint by its owner, you know that "the tumor has what it takes to be clinical." Otherwise, the tumor would never have surfaced. That is the central paradigm of an evolutionary process. If you move detection earlier in time, you move detection earlier in an evolutionary process. We can illustrate this by looking at *Homo sapiens*, a very successful species. Move back in evolutionary time, and you find surprisingly many hominids, all now extinct. They didn't have what it takes. Only one sequence of hominids succeeded in acquiring sufficient (energetically very costly) brain power without dying out. If there are so few fossil hominid remnants, it is because the route of investing in brainpower was a very risky one. Post hoc, it is easy to identify the successful species line, but it would have been utterly impossible at the time to predict which of the hominids would be successful. Similarly, if you move back in tumor history, it is increasingly difficult to predict which cell line will be aggressive and which not.

Lead time is the additional length of survival with disease brought about by earlier diagnosis. Lead time comes at the cost of survival free of disease, before cancer diagnosis. To give an example: without screening, a patient might be diagnosed with clinical breast cancer at age 55 and die at age 60. But with screening, she might be diagnosed at age 53 but still die at age 60. Her "survival" subsequent to screening improves by two years, but this is because her life expectancy free of disease decreases by two years. We see, therefore, that a result of screening survival after diagnosis becomes longer but the screened person may die at the same point in time. In those cancers where incidence increases with increasing age, lead time by earlier diagnosis causes an apparent increase in age-adjusted cancer incidence.

Another problem is that some tumors grow rapidly, others grow slowly. This can be likened to taking a trip on a slow train; it will pick up only those passengers who are not in a hurry, while those who are in a rush will have left to go by a fast car. This is called length time.[10,11] Screening will pick up the slow-growing tumors (and hence the ones with good prognosis), but will miss the rapidly growing ones. That means it will detect the tumor, but the tumor has already metastasized. Any detectable tumor has existed for years, and if the cell line is inclined to metastasize, that line has had ample time to do so before detection of the lesion is even possible. Finally, the natural history of screen-detected tumors cannot be predicted: earlier in the carcinogenic process, more tumors "don't have what it takes." They look malignant, but have not yet acquired the potential for invasive growth. This is called "pseudodiagnosis."[10,11] Lead time, length time, and pseudodiagnosis all cause increases of iatrogenic cancer morbidity. Screening tends to pick up the "losers:" tumors that stay for prolonged periods in a detectable phase and are therefore not particularly aggressive. If you waited for a clinical diagnosis, many of these tumors would still have been curable as they are not aggressive. Screening therefore tends to miss the "winners:" the tumors that stay only for a short period in a detectable phase before metastasis. In these very aggressive tumors, even when detected, metastasis has already happened before the tumor was detectable.

As a consequence of lead time, length time, and pseudodiagnosis, cancer "incidence" (I prefer the word "detection" as incidence is unobservable) jumps up and survival of patients with screen-detected tumors is very high. These are all happy patients, broadcasting the news of their salvation.

Attributing the cause of death

The aim of cancer screening is, of course, to decrease mortality. But another problem emerges here. People at high risk for a specific cancer (because of genetic or familial reasons, or with precancerous or pre-existing disease) should not be included in population screening programs as they need clinical follow-up. A woman with breast cancer should not be referred to a population screening program for follow-up. After excluding the high-risk group, the remaining eligible population is at low risk. At the same time, cancer incidence is high in an aging population with increasing morbidity and mortality from other causes. In the Swedish breast cancer screening cohorts, at the end of follow-up 20% were dead, but only 0.4% died of breast cancer, and screening apparently reduced mortality by 0.1%.[4] How confident can you be that a decline of 0.1% in a total of 20% is not balanced by an increase of 0.1% somewhere else? Assigning cause of death in screening trials is therefore of crucial importance. But a monocausal classification of cause of death ignores the complex web of causation leading to death in older people with concurrent morbidity and competing risks of death.[5]

The first bias in allocation of cause of death arises as the information in the screened and the unscreened is asymmetric. In the screened cohorts, more women know for a longer time that they have breast cancer. If they die of a poorly identified disorder, a handy cause of death is available. This, of course, would increase apparent cancer mortality in the screened group. This bias has been coined "sticky bias."[5] The diagnosis of breast cancer sticks, and may replace other causes of death. However, there are many more people diagnosed and treated in the screened arm. The stress of having been given a diagnosis of a potentially fatal disorder followed by treatment (surgical intervention, and radiotherapy or chemotherapy) may cause death from other causes, notably cardiovascular disease. For example, a 64-year-old woman with diabetes and pre-existing angina is found with a small tumor and operated on. She dies two days later from a heart attack. That is obviously not a cancer-related death. But it might be a screening-related death, as without screening and the stress of diagnosis and treatment, she might not have had a heart attack. Furthermore, in the 1980s, the years of the trials, radiotherapy of the left breast was complicated by damage of the heart muscle. So the cause of death could have been related to the process of screening and treating, while not being attributable to breast cancer. This bias is called "slippery" as the diagnosis tends to slip away.[5]

Of course, a cancer diagnosis may be simply misallocated. In the analysis of the Swedish breast cancer screening trials, there was an apparent decline of breast cancer mortality but no apparent change in all-cancer mortality. Re-analysis of the Ostergötland data from the most powered Two County Trial (Ostergötland and Kopparberg; the trials were merged) showed little change at all in breast cancer mortality in the screened group. Unfortunately, the investigators of Kopparberg have refused to cooperate, something that does nothing to inspire confidence in the reliability of their conclusions.

Deliberate bias in publications

The authors of the recent meta-analysis (the Nyström group), who re-analyzed the Ostergötland data, did not research the reasons for the inconsistent findings in Ostergötland. These inconsistencies were only commented on as a reason to include the poor Ostergötland data. Indeed, the meagre results weakened the overall effect. This is highly remarkable as in the original study a strong decrease in breast cancer mortality was "observed." You might want to know the reason why the strong decrease disappeared after re-analysis: it would enlighten the reader about the process of allocation of causes of death in screening trials. It is even more remarkable that the authors of Kopparberg are still allowed to publish findings of this trial (or to publish at all) as they refused to cooperate with the re-analysis and to make their data available for independent scrutiny. In the light of the supposed large decrease in breast cancer mortality but the complete absence of any decrease in all-cancer mortality, an independent audit of the causes of death of the participants seems warranted. The very positive results of the Two County Trial pushed many countries into establishing organized population breast cancer screening; it is a shame that so many clouds are allowed to remain over these results.

In the papers from the breast screening trials absolute risks are hard to find, and numbers needed to screen are never included. The much touted relative risk reduction of 20% implies that you will need 10 000 years of follow-up in order to prevent one death from breast cancer. In papers from the breast screening trials, no incidence, treatment, and complication rates have been published. This allows the lie to persist that more screening participants are treated with less invasive treatments. The Danish Cochrane center found that after breast cancer screening, the absolute risk of any cancer treatment increased by 0.2%, and the absolute risk of a mastectomy increased by 0.1%.[12] This causes a slight decrease in the relative proportion of invasive treatments in the screened arm, but an absolute increase in the numbers of the women to be treated invasively.

Cancer screening trials seem to give only the good news (decreases in a mortality of a specific cancer mortality), but do not give the bad news (increases in cancer treatment).

Societal processes in cancer screening

Sometimes a cancer is not detected at screening but appears during the interval between screening rounds. Such cancers are called "interval cancers." The victims are not happy customers as they had believed that they were free of cancer. They sometimes take the radiologist to court. In the USA cases involving breast cancer are the second most common cause of malpractice litigation, the leading allegation being failure to diagnose.[13] This pushes doctors on to the defensive: fearful of missing something, they tend to be more "sensitive" and less specific in the interpretation of screening tests. The price to pay is increasing rates of false positives. In breast cancer screening in the Netherlands, the detection rates of breast cancer during screening were close to 2% (implying 1% false positives). In the USA they are 6% (5% false positives) and in Belgium they can increase to 12% (11% false positives).[14] The unavoidable occurrence of interval cancers keeps the screening system under continuous pressure which results in more overdiagnosis: false positives are in general happy costumers, only the false negatives complain about medical malpractice.

Demonstration of an economic model

A well-known cancer screening model is the Dutch MISCAN; this can simulate individual disease histories.[6] The input is very complex while the output is rarely if ever shown in terms of age- and screening-dependent rates of cancer incidence and mortality. Publication of all relevant rates of incidence and mortality by age and by time since intervention (both observed and as modeled) should be a golden rule in evaluating health economic papers. It would be immediately apparent that the core "results" of many models are, in reality, arguable assumptions. Nobody can predict the dynamic consequences of these many assumptions in complex models. Age- and time-dependent rates allow the reader to judge the face validity of the results. The common lack of published incidence and mortality rates in simulated screened and unscreened populations over the entire life course might be inspired by fear of being exposed as mathematical emperors without empirical clothes. In a nutshell, this complex model is an elaborate exercise in recycling simple and simplistic concepts. Figure 11.1 simulates the effect of screening on breast cancer incidence and mortality; it illustrates some of the assumptions that seem innocuous but have far-reaching effects.

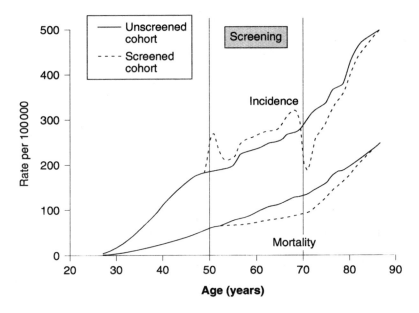

Figure 11.1 Results that show the effect of screening on incidence and mortality from breast cancer in a computer simulation model. Women received either screening from age 50 to 70 (dashed line) or no screening (continuous line).

I will start by describing the cancer incidence in the screened cohort. At the first round of screening, a firm "bulge" is observed. The first round picks up all the detectable tumors that might have existed for years. The subsequent dip is a consequence of exhaustion of this pool. The steady increase thereafter is generated by the underlying true rise in cancer incidence. After stopping screening at age 70, it will take time to "refill" the exhausted numbers of clinical tumors. Indeed, in the model all tumors detected are clinical tumors. The area under the incidence line is equal in the screened and unscreened cohorts: the increase in incidence during screening is exactly the same as the decrease after screening.

The risk of mortality due to breast cancer in the screened group decreases gradually to a level 35% lower than in the unscreened subjects. As the screened tumors are all potentially lethal, the mortality decrease shows how screening picks up tumors between ages 50 and 70 that would have been lethal between ages 70 and 88. The lowered mortality continues for the rest of the person's life (here the cohorts were cut artificially at age 88).

As each case of terminal cancer is expensive, the lowered mortality saves much money. In the model, screening will generate net savings as small tumors detected early and treated more conservatively in the screened cohort appear years later as large tumors treated more aggressively in the unscreened cohort. That is also the reason for the long duration of the mortality decline.

This simple figure unveils the simplistic assumptions of linearity that make screening appear to be highly cost-effective. Earlier treatment does not increase costs. Rather, as screening allows diagnosis to be made some years earlier, it necessarily improves prognosis and saves costs. The synthetic screened cohort experiences no overdiagnosis. The falling incidence after age 70 is sheer imagination. The authors of this model were instrumental in having the end of screening postponed to age 75, and proposed to continue up to age 80. In countries with long-standing screening programs (Sweden, Denmark, Netherlands), the increases in incidence were 40% to 50%, and there is no reason that might have caused this except for increased detection by screening. Mortality decreases are hard to interpret. The secular trends in the European breast cancer mortality decrease have been credited to breast cancer screening, but this ignores the widespread introduction of tamoxifen for cancer treatment.[15] Indeed, breast cancer mortality has decreased in all European countries, whether screening programs exist or not.

Breast cancer screening: conclusions

An economic analysis of screening trials evaluates the costs and effects of a hypothesis. Other hypotheses will yield different conclusions. Cost-effectiveness analyses cloud the main issues. With the present epidemiological tools, we cannot determine beyond a reasonable doubt that cancer screening is effective. If we screen 1000 people for 10 years, on average one will benefit and many will be harmed. Indeed, reassurance in cancer screening is false reassurance as interval cancers emerge after screening, and if timely diagnosis is important, it is in clinically apparent cancers as these "have what it takes" to be lethal. By becoming clinically apparent, they have demonstrated their malignant potential. In aging societies, confronted with an enormous and increasing availability of truly effective healthcare technology for persons with diseases and complaints, the provision of costly screening of limited effectiveness for healthy people at low risk should be reconsidered.

Screening for other types of cancer

This chapter is intended to be general, focusing on processes in cancer screening and how they are manipulated by health economic models. Most examples are from breast cancer screening but most types of cancer screening have more or less the same trade-offs of harms and benefits.

If we disregard the doubt about the validity of cause of death classification, breast cancer screening yields benefits for one in 1000 women. In the real life of day-to-day clinical practice, for every death prevented some five screened women are harmed by unnecessary treatment and a further 25 will have a biopsy.

Cervical cancer screening is likely more effective than is the case with breast cancer, but it is a rare disorder, at least in wealthy market economies. You need to screen 1000 women for 20 years to prevent one death. These numbers will go up further by a factor of four in the generation born after 1970, a consequence of HIV-AIDS, steeply decreased gonorrhea rates, and expected decreases in human papilloma virus (HPV) transmission. Overdiagnosis and overtreatment are enormous, but treatment is generally limited and mild. Vaccination against HPV, one of the causative agents of cervical cancer, is promising.

The benefits of colorectal cancer screening with effective methods are also around one in 1000. The major disadvantage is the high induced demand for colonoscopy. This may influence availability for patients with complaints. Again, it is important to note that timely diagnosis is most important in cancer that shows clinically detectable symptoms. It is close to medical negligence to consider colorectal cancer screening in a country that has apparent capacity problems and waiting lists for colonoscopy. Screening will increase capacity problems, waiting lists, and treatment delays for real cancer patients.

Prostate cancer screening is medical malpractice. There is no evidence that screening yields any benefits, and if it yields benefits, these will be very small. Prostate cancer is an old man's disease. In the Netherlands, the probability of dying of prostate cancer before age 75 is 1.25%. The mean age at death from prostate cancer is six years older than the mean age at death in the population. Populations eligible for screening (and hence without increased risk of prostate cancer) will be at even lower risk of death.

Induction of harm by screening for prostate cancer is not a probability but a certainty. All cancers manifest occult disease, disease that looks malignant but with an uncertain evolution. However, in prostate cancer, prevalence of occult disease is very high, reaching 40% and more in healthy middle-aged males. This occult disease is revealed by screening and leads to mutilating interventions without clinical benefit. Screening is carried out by measuring the blood level of prostate-specific antigen level (PSA). It indicates a risk in much the same way as high blood pressure indicates a risk for stroke. Many men with a persistent low PSA still have prostate cancer, while many men with high PSA do not have prostate cancer. This leads to high rates of prostate biopsies. This procedure is a lousy confirmation test: a negative test does not exclude the presence of prostate cancer. Repeated biopsies are therefore required and these have their own complication rates. Most small tumors grow exceedingly slowly or not at all. In occult tumors detected by screening with PSA, there is no evidence that treatment is better than watchful waiting. In palpable small tumors (not screen-detected) surgical intervention produces a risk of death from prostate cancer that is only slightly lower than that seen with watchful waiting. It takes eight years to detect any benefit: limited life expectancy among older males further reduces benefit. The complications of treatment are horrendous, with close to 90% of treated males becoming impotent and 50% suffering incontinence after radical prostatectomy – this in centers of excellence participating in screening trials. After radiotherapy, prevalence of incontinence and impotence is lower, but radiation colitis is a frequent and disabling sequel.

Those who die of prostate cancer have had, in general, the advantage of a long life in above average health. But if they had been screened, they would risk incontinence and impotence, as well as losing many years free of worries. Moreover, it will be impossible to prove that prostate cancer screening added a single day to their life. The problems of screening trials are considerably worse with prostate cancer than in other cancer screening as the hazards of co-morbidity and competing mortality are very high in older men, the target of screening.

Screening has brought about a jump in the "incidence" of prostate cancer in the USA and most countries of Europe, but without any apparent change in mortality. Putting it another way, the rise in prostate cancer "incidence" is associated with a dramatic – and spurious – rise in survival rates; this illustrates the guiding principles of preventive quackery: frighten people and talk them into disease. Treating nonexistent disease in healthy people is much more rewarding than treating truly ill people: they will be happy survivors of a dreadful disease, saved by prevention.[16]

References

1   Schneider BL and Kulesz-Martin M (2004) Destructive cycles: the role of genomic instability and adaptation in carcinogenesis. *Carcinogenesis*. **25**: 2033–44.
2   Malins DC, Johnson PM, Barker EA, Polissar NL, Wheeler TM and Anderson KM (2003) Cancer-related changes in prostate DNA as men age and early identification of metastasis in primary prostate tumors. *Proc Natl Acad Sci USA*. **100**: 5401–6.
3   Franco OH, Peeters A, Looman CW and Bonneux L (2005) Cost effectiveness of statins in coronary heart disease. *J Epidemiol Community Health*. **59**: 927–33.
4   Nyström L, Andersson I, Bjurstam N, Frisell J, Nordenskjöld B and Rutqvist LE (2002) Long-term effects of mammography screening: updated overview of the Swedish randomised trials. *Lancet*. **359**: 909–19.
5   Black WC, Haggstrom DA and Welch H (2002) All cause mortality in randomized trials of cancer screening. *J Natl Cancer Inst*. **94**: 167–73.
6   Habbema JD, van Oortmarssen GJ, Lubbe JT and van der Maas PJ (1985) The MISCAN simulation program for the evaluation of screening for disease. *Comput Methods Programs Biomed*. **20**:79–93.
7   van der Maas PJ, de Koning HJ, van Ineveld BM, van Oortmarssen GJ, Habbema JD and Lubbe KT (1989) The cost-effectiveness of breast cancer screening. *Int J Cancer*. **43**: 1055–60.
8   Malins DC, Polissar NL, Schaefer S, Su Y and Vinson M (1998) A unified theory of carcinogenesis based on order–disorder transitions in DNA structure as studied in the human ovary and breast. *Proc Natl Acad Sci USA*. **95**: 7637–42.
9   Mandelblatt J, Saha S, Teutsch S *et al.* (2003) The cost-effectiveness of screening mammography beyond age 65 years: a systematic review for the U.S. Preventive Services Task Force. *Ann Intern Med*. **139**: 835–42.
10 Cole P and Morrison AS (1980) Basic issues in population screening for cancer. *J Natl Cancer Inst*. **64**: 1263–72.
11 Black WC and Welch HG (1993) Advances in diagnostic imaging and overestimations of disease prevalence and the benefits of therapy. *N Engl J Med*. **328**: 1237–43.
12 Olsen O and Gøtzsche PG (2001) Cochrane review on screening for breast cancer with mammography. *Lancet*. **358**: 1340–2.
13 Guthrie TH (1999) Breast cancer litigation: an update with practice guidelines. *Breast J*. **5**: 335–9.
14 Paulus D, Mambourg F and Bonneux L (2005) *Breast Cancer Screening*. Belgian Health Care Knowledge Center, Brussels.
15 Bonneux L (2003) Mortality reduction by breast cancer screening. *Lancet*. **362**: 245.
16 Romains J (1922) *Knock, ou le Triomphe de la Médecine*. © 1924 Par Gallimard. Impression Bussiere a St-Amand (Cher).

Chapter 12

The Canadian National Breast Screening Study: science meets controversy

Cornelia J. Baines

Please note that the following is a short version of this chapter, the full version can be found on the Radcliffe website (www.radcliffe-oxford.com/medicalspending).

Introduction

The Canadian National Breast Screening Study (CNBSS) included two individually randomized controlled trials of breast screening to evaluate the efficacy of screening. The goal of screening is to achieve sufficiently early detection of a disease, such as breast cancer, so that deaths are prevented. The questions posed in the CNBSS precisely reflected US recommendations developed by a National Cancer Institute/ American Cancer Society Working Group[1] after careful scrutiny of then-available screening data. Thus the first Canadian trial asked: In women aged 40–49, what is the benefit of combined screening with mammography (MA) and clinical breast examination (CBE) compared to no screening at all? The second one asked: In women aged 50–59 what is the incremental benefit of MA over and above CBE? Seven-year,[2,3] 10.5-year,[4] and 13-year[5,6] CNBSS mortality results have been published.

The CNBSS began screening women aged 40–59 in January 1980. Women who were pregnant, had a previous history of breast cancer, or had had a mammogram in the preceding 12 months were excluded. All received annual mailed questionnaires, either over four years (for the women in the first two-thirds recruited) or three years (for the later recruits). All received breast self-examination instructions. For 50 430 women aged 40–49 on entry, the CNBSS compared breast cancer mortality in those receiving annual MA and CBE, with mortality in those who received a single CBE on entry and thereafter reverted to community care. For 39 405 women aged 50–59 on entry, the CNBSS compared mortality in those receiving annual MA and CBE, with mortality in those receiving annual CBE. Women were assigned to MA and comparison groups by a systematic randomization procedure applied to each woman individually. Randomization is important to avoid bias.

The point at which randomization occurred in CNBSS became a contentious issue, although at the time the study was designed, it seemed well justified. Randomization of all 90 000 women was implemented in the 15 national centers by the center coordinators *after* the nurse-examiner had performed the entry CBE. The reason for this sequence was two-fold. It was believed that the nurse-examiner might be influenced if she knew that a woman had already been assigned to the MA group. Thus, if the examiner were uncertain as to whether a CBE was abnormal, she might not designate it as abnormal if she could "rely" on MA to settle the matter. What was wanted was a "call" on the CBE uninfluenced by any knowledge that MA was to follow. This was information that could only be gained on the first screening visit because thereafter the woman's assignment to MA would be known. The second reason related to informed consent. By 1980, this was required in randomized controlled trials in Canada, for both those receiving the intervention and for control subjects. This required all participants to come and register for the trial and sign informed consent forms at the screening centers. However, it seemed an unacceptable inconvenience to have the 25 000 women aged 40–49 who would be randomized to the control group come to the center only to be sent on their way. Therefore, identical self-reported information was collected from the two groups.

The CNBSS differs markedly from other screening trials. It was the first trial specifically designed to examine whether screening women aged 40–49 was effective. Only CNBSS controls received single (40–49-year-olds) or annual (50–59-year-olds) CBE screening. Only CNBSS controls submitted information annually. Only the CNBSS had a structured audit of MA.[7] Only in the CNBSS were tissue sections from all breast surgical procedures reviewed by reference pathologists and compared to diagnoses reached by the community pathologists.[2,3] Trial conduct was monitored by an international Policy Advisory Group. Uniquely, the CNBSS and Health Insurance Plan of New York (HIP) Study appointed external expert panels, blind to screening status, to determine whether breast cancer was the actual cause of death in women known to have breast cancer. The CNBSS panel also determined by examining hospital records whether breast cancer was the actual cause of death in women with death certificate diagnoses of lung and liver cancer. And the CNBSS was one of only three screening studies (along with the HIP Study and the Malmo study) to employ individual, as opposed to cluster, randomization.

This chapter first discusses the CNBSS in the context of criticisms pertaining to randomization, MA, "contamination," and results, with reference to other screening trials. Second, it reviews the mortality paradox wherein screened women aged 40–49 are more likely to die of breast cancer in the first years after screening is initiated compared to unscreened control women. Third, it examines whether women who currently seek MA screening are completely informed and, if not, why not. Finally, it speculates on the nature of the breast screening controversy.

Conclusion

For more than two decades some have promoted screening breast cancer by employing questionable tactics.[8-11] Such tactics, combined with appealing promises, may sway the media and the public, but they do not resolve socio-scientific controversies and it is highly questionable that women are truly benefiting. It is useful to look at the screening controversy from the context of the "Four I's" as shown below, but the same method can be applied to many other socio-scientific controversies.

First the Idea

The idea that early detection must be useful for controlling cancer is intuitively indisputable. The benefit has not yet been clearly established for breast cancer, and one must consider whether the early detection currently being achieved is not early enough.

Second the Individual

The individuals in the breast screening controversy are women and their doctors. The women are afraid of breast cancer and want mammography to reassure themselves. The doctors may know the limitations of MA screening, but they also know that delayed detection is a major cause of medico-legal litigation in the USA. They really have little opportunity to practice evidence-based screening.

Third the Interests

(As in, conflict of interest.) Breast screening yields revenue to radiologists, to surgeons and pathologists, and to the manufacturers of MA and ultrasound units, film, film processing chemicals, and biopsy equipment. It is interesting that internists (as reflected by their professional associations) have tended not to endorse screening as rapidly as other specialist organizations. A few years ago the *Economist*[12] said very bluntly that the controversy was driven by professional and corporate greed.

Fourth, the Institutions

Among the strongest promoters of screening has been the American College of Radiology, which has been virulent in its denunciation of the CNBSS. It has powerful resources to spread its message. Governments are potential sources of objective guidelines, but they sustain tremendous political pressures, all of which were shown dramatically following the 1997 consensus conference when the US Senate, believing it knew more about screening policy than the convened NIH panel, unanimously overturned its recommendations.[13]

The International Agency for Research on Cancer (IARC) Working Group on Breast Cancer Screening recently concluded that evidence supporting MA screening (compared to no screening) in women aged 40–49 is inconsistent and statistically not significant. For women aged 50–59 the evidence is consistent and statistically significant.[14] However, CNBSS results for women aged 50–59 show that while MA detects far more breast cancers and smaller cancers than CBE, at 13-year follow-up, annual MA plus CBE compared to CBE alone does not reduce breast cancer deaths.[4]

New and better approaches are needed to "control" breast cancer. In the meantime it seems reasonable for women aged 40–49 not to accept MA screening. However, the situation is different for women aged 50–59. Screening trials that compared MA screening to no screening have shown modest reductions in breast cancer mortality accruing from MA. Thus is it reasonable for women in this age group to accept screening provided they are assured of technically excellent mammograms. Where screening MA is not available or not wanted, high quality clinical breast examination is likely to be useful, provided diagnostic MA facilities are available.

References

1 Working Group (1979) Report of the Working Group to Review the National Cancer Institute–American Cancer Society Breast Cancer Detection Demonstration Projects. *J Natl Cancer Inst.* **62**: 639–709.

2 Miller AB, Baines CJ, To T *et al.* (1992) Canadian National Breast Screening Study – 1. Breast cancer detection and death rates among women aged 40–49 years. *Can Med Assoc J.* **147**: 1459–76. Correction: *Can Med Assoc J.* (1993) **148**: 718.

3 Miller AB, Baines CJ, To T *et al.* (1992) Canadian National Breast Screening Study – 2. Breast cancer detection and death rates among women aged 50–59 years. *Can Med Assoc J.* **147**: 1477–88. Correction: *Can Med Assoc J.* (1993) **148**: 718.

4 Miller AB, To T, Baines CJ and Wall C (1997) The Canadian Breast Screening Study: update on breast cancer mortality. *Monogr Natl Cancer Inst.* **22**: 37–41.

5 Miller AB, To T, Baines CJ and Wall C (2000) Canadian National Breast Screening Study – 2: 13-year results of a randomized trial in women aged 50–59 years. *J Natl Cancer Inst.* **92**: 1490–9.

6 Miller AB, To T, Baines CJ and Wall C (2002) The Canadian National Breast Screening Study – 1: Breast cancer mortality after 11–16 years follow-up. A randomized trial of screening mammography in women age 40 to 49 years. *Ann Intern Med.* **137**: 305–12.

7 Baines CJ, McFarlane DV and Wall C (1986) Audit procedures in the National Breast Screening Study: mammography interpretation. *Can Assoc Radiol J.* **37**: 256–60.

8 Baines CJ (1994) The Canadian National Breast Screening Study: a perspective on criticism. *Ann Intern Med.* **120**: 326–34.

9 Crewdson J (2000) In Sweden, decades of mammograms barely cut deaths. *Chicago Tribune,* March 18.

10 Taubes G (1997) How one radiologist turns up the heat. *Science.* **275**: 1057.

11 Kopans DB (2002) Needless confusion over mammograms. *Boston Globe,* January 1: A19.

12 Economist (1997) Screening for cancer. *Economist* **343**: 19.

13 Ernster VL (1997) Mammographic screening for women aged 40 through 49: a guidelines saga and a clarion call for informed decision making. *Am J Public Health.* **7**: 1103–6.

14 IARC (2002) *Handbooks of Cancer Prevention. Vol. 7. Breast Cancer Screening.* IARC Press, Lyon.

Chapter 13

Screening for breast cancer: benefits versus costs

Andrew Thompson and Norman J. Temple

Introduction

When we look at various medical procedures they often appear to be tremendous boons to society, or at least at first glance they have that appearance. But, as we saw with the use of statins, even when a treatment promises to prevent one-third of future cases of a common disease, it may still be, in reality, of quite limited value.

It is well known that for several types of cancer early detection facilitates their treatment. It seems self-evident therefore that screening for cancer is a very sensible thing to do. But not everything that seems self-evident stands up to close examination. In light of this we will carefully evaluate the case for screening for cancer. Chapter 11 has already covered much of the ground. In Chapter 12 Cornelia Barnes reviewed the findings from the two Canadian screening trials for breast cancer. These indicated that screening is of no value for women aged 40–49 and there are question marks as to its value for women aged over 50. The Canadian trials were conducted with great care and the findings are as reliable as those from any of the other trials. Nevertheless, the unwelcome findings from these trials generated a hostile response from some quarters of the medical establishment. These attacks were often based on a distortion of the facts and her experiences are illuminating as a description of this.

In this chapter the focus is again on breast cancer, and in the next we look at cervical cancer. In doing these analyses we will strive to look at the "big picture." This means not only evaluating claims for the efficacy of screening (i.e. cancer deaths prevented) but also examining adverse effects, most notably the harm caused by false positives.

We will also attempt to determine how much it costs to generate one quality-adjusted life year (QALY) by screening. As explained in Chapter 1, the QALY is the most appropriate measure as it takes into account the fact that the extra years of life are often of reduced quality, either as a direct result of the medical intervention or simply because some or most of those years occur in older age. But only by making a careful cost assessment can we reliably determine if the expenditure of large sums of public money for mass screening is justified.

We have disregarded prostate cancer because the value of screening by the digital-rectal examination (DRE) and the prostate-specific antigen level (PSA) has been shown, in numerous papers in medical journals, to be outweighed by the harm that results from the treatment of positive findings.[1,2] This harm includes marked increases in impotence and incontinence in return for very little, if any, extension of life. Many men who have been "cured" of prostate cancer may find that they have been handed a pyrrhic victory.

What is the effectiveness of mammography?

It is almost impossible for the average woman to be unaware that the official voice of medical wisdom strongly encourages women to have regular mammograms. The theory is that this procedure will detect breast cancer at an early stage when treatment is likely to be more successful. There is debate over whether screening should commence at age 40 or 50 and whether mammography (MA) should be performed every year or every two years.

That is what medical orthodoxy has been preaching since the 1980s. But there is another side of the story. Here we will examine three crucial questions.

- Is MA really as effective as its proponents claim?
- What harm does MA cause?
- What is the real cost of MA (how much does it cost in order to prolong life)?

The conventional view of MA is exemplified in an overview of several Swedish trials. This found that at ages 40–69 MA achieves a 21% reduction in risk of death from breast cancer.[3] Similarly, in 2002 the US Preventive Services Task Force reviewed the efficacy of MA.[4,5] The task force found all four Swedish trials and the New York trial to be of "fair" quality, the two Canadian trials of fair or better, and the Edinburgh trial of "poor" (not useable) quality. After correcting for some flaws in the trials, its mathematical combination of the trials indicated that MA produces a statistically significant reduction in death from breast cancer. The reduction was small, requiring 1792 women in their forties and 1224 women in the combined 40–74 age range to have MA for 14 years in order for one breast cancer death to be prevented. Nevertheless, they concluded that although the data supporting MA for women aged 40–49 was not strong, this group, plus older women, should have annual or biennial screening.

But there are those who have voiced serious doubts as to the reliability of these findings. In Chapter 11 Luc Bonneux reviewed aspects of the evidence concerning MA and identified various problems. Peter Gøtzsche and Ole Olsen[6] from Denmark reviewed the eight trials which provide the case for the effectiveness of MA and found only three of them were sufficiently free from serious faults to be trustworthy. These three, the two Canadian trials and the Malmö Swedish trial, found no preventive effect for MA. The other six had numerous faults, the most serious being possibly biased randomization of subjects into the MA intervention and control groups. The paper by Olsen and Gotzsche lead to a storm of controversy in the medical press. There was a vigorous defense of the faulted trials by their authors and various commentators. Olsen and Gøtsche then wrote a second review,[7] which confirmed and extended their conclusion that there is no statistically significant difference in favor of MA in terms of prevention of death from breast cancer. However, to complete their report they did a mathematical analysis including all but the two most flawed trials. This found much the same small advantage as the task force's analysis.

One of the criticisms made by Olsen and Gotsche[8] is that breast cancer mortality is an unreliable outcome, being subject to misclassification of cause of death. Such an error could completely change the results. This problem was discussed in Chapter 2. Olsen and Gotsche noted that, despite the attempted masking of group membership, review committees attributed more uncertain causes of deaths as being due to breast cancer in the control group than in the MA group. In their opinion, only evidence of an actual difference in all-cause mortality is the crucial test to prove the efficacy of MA, and such evidence is lacking. Unfortunately, trying to prove that MA leads to a decrease in all-cause mortality would require trials of enormous size (and enormous cost).

Now, it would be easy to dismiss Olsen and Gotsche as having a rather extreme interpretation of the evidence. But these investigators are far from alone. Indeed, some highly credible experts have voiced similar views. We can point to Michael Baum,[9] who was principal investigator of the largest group for breast cancer trials in Europe. He highlighted significant errors in the design and analysis of the trials. Likewise, Richard Horton,[10] Editor of the *Lancet*, stated in an editorial: "At present there is no reliable evidence from large randomised trials to support screening mammography programmes."

The controversy over MA was examined by the expert panel that advised the US National Cancer Institute (NCI). The experts decided to revise their original draft and concluded that there was insufficient evidence that mammograms prevent breast cancer deaths.[11] This was reported in the *New York Times* in January 2002, along with an editorial that described MA as "so strongly endorsed by the cancer establishment, and has become such a significant source of revenue ... for many hospitals and doctors, that it may be difficult to excise without overwhelming evidence that it is dangerous."[12] But the NCI rejected the findings of its own advisory panel and issued a press release repeating the old wisdom that women, including those aged in their forties, should be screened every one to two years by MA.

The vast majority of women have been convinced by the massive marketing of MA that they should follow the recommendations of the "experts." Third party payers will continue to include MA in their benefits because, even if they have doubts of its efficacy, they know that their subscribers might desert them if they try to drop it. Governments will also continue to pay for it because its members do not want to risk losing favor with the medical establishment or any sizeable segment of the electorate.

In short, the evidence to date indicates, if one accepts less than good trial data, a tiny proportion of women will be less likely to die of breast cancer if they have MA, but not that those who are thus prevented from dying from this disease will necessarily live longer. However, MA is an entrenched practice that will continue to be highly promoted unless new evidence is offered that casts substantial doubt on its overall benefit.

Adverse effects of mammography

We shall now look at the physical and psychological harm resulting from MA. This harm begins with the process of MA itself. It is painful to some women since it requires that each breast be forcibly compressed. Another kind of harm is the surgical excision, radiographic treatment, and breast reconstruction surgery that is undertaken when women are diagnosed as having ductal cancer *in situ* (DCIS). This condition is difficult to diagnose and is not necessarily a cancer,[13] often recurs,[14] and has never been proven to result in more breast cancer deaths.[15,16] However, it results in one in every 65 women in the USA having surgery to excise it, given current medical practice.[16] MA does not, in itself, cause this surgery – this is due to the advice of the involved medical personnel – but without MA over 90% of DCIS diagnoses would not be made and those women would not have lumpectomy or mastectomy, radiation therapy, and the associated procedures.

The most prevalent type of harm occurs from false positives. This is when cancer is suspected of being present, but further procedures, such as another mammogram and biopsy of suspicious tissue, find no cancer. Here, the final reassurance is real but the initial anxiety may be intense and prolonged. If women have biennial screening for 10 years, then about 23% of them will have at least one false positive.[4] This suggests that, for every woman whose death from breast cancer is prevented, roughly 500 will have a disturbing phone call followed by further investigation. This is a negative result of MA that should not be ignored.

How much does all this cost?

Let us now attempt to calculate how much it costs to prevent one death from breast cancer using MA. As in other chapters we will attempt to answer this question by estimating how many dollars must be spent in order to generate one QALY. Despite the weaknesses in the evidence we will make this calculation on the assumption that MA is indeed effective. The more enthusiastic supporters claim that MA reduces risk of death from breast cancer by 20% to 30%, or even more. We shall base our calculation on the viewpoint of the US Preventive Services Task Force of MA.[4] As stated earlier the task force estimated that 1224 women in the age range 40–74 would require mammograms for 14 years in order to prevent one death from breast cancer (i.e. number needed to screen [NNS] is 1224; NNS is equivalent to number needed to treat [NNT]). We shall assume that the women in the MA groups had an average of seven mammograms during the 14-year follow-up period. What then is the cost to prevent one death that is diagnosed as being due to breast cancer?

The average cost of a mammogram is $125.[17] A review of 10 consecutive years of files in an health maintenance organization of 2400 women between the ages of 40 and 69 at study entry revealed that for every $100 spent for MA, $33 was spent for follow-up of false positive results.[18] This raises the cost of each mammogram to $167. This amount times seven (the average number of mammograms) times 1224 (NNS) results in a total cost of $1.43 million.

To convert this cost into QALYs we need an estimate of how many years of extra life are generated when death from breast cancer is prevented by MA. As pointed out earlier, there is no hard evidence that such prevention actually prolongs lives. However, we will assume for this exercise that there is indeed some extension of life.

The usual assumption is that the women will live out a full lifespan. How many years is that? According to Canadian data, for women who died from breast cancer between ages 45 and 74, the mean age at death is approximately 62.[19] The life expectancy for an average American woman at age 62 is 84.[20] So the maximum theoretically possible added years of life would be around 22 (i.e. 84 minus 62), other things being equal. But other things are seldom equal. Some of the lifestyle factors that contribute to having breast cancer – such as obesity, lack of exercise, and excessive alcohol consumption – also contribute to other diseases. For this reason, women who develop breast cancer probably have, on average, a lower life expectancy than other women. A more realistic estimate of life extension, therefore, is 19 years (rather than 22). These last years are not apt to be of high quality, perhaps a quality of 0.8 on the QALY scale of zero to 1.0, with 1.0 being perfect health. Each death from breast cancer prevented therefore generates, on average, roughly 15.2 QALYs. From this we conclude that the cost per QALY is approximately $94 000 (i.e. $1.43 million divided by 15.2).

Now we freely admit that this figure is a rather crude estimate. However, even if the correct figure is appreciably lower, this cost analysis strongly suggests that a screening MA program is an unacceptably expensive medical expenditure. We base this on our proposed cost limit, as stated in Chapter 1, of $50 000 per QALY as a medium-term goal, and $27 000 per QALY as both an ideal limit and a longer-term goal. In reality, there are reasons that suggest that we may well have *underestimated* the true cost of MA as the claimed benefits of MA may have been exaggerated, as we discussed earlier. In addition, false positives cause real harm; striking a fear of death into as many as 30% of healthy women into order to save a tiny number is a real cost, albeit one that is impossible to quantify.

Conclusions

The medical establishment in the USA strongly recommends screening for breast cancer with MA for women aged 40–74. The best way to determine the value of this recommendation is to look at the overall picture of the balance of benefits and harms to the women involved. The estimates based on long-term trials indicate that the benefit is quite modest: only one woman aged 40–74 out of every 1220 or so can be expected to not die of breast cancer because of MA. However, there are good reasons to suspect that the benefits of MA have been exaggerated. The one piece of truly hard evidence would be a study showing that MA lowers all-cause mortality, but such evidence is lacking.

Counterbalancing any deaths from breast cancer avoided, MA indisputably causes harm, most notably from false positives that lead to additional diagnostic procedures and anxiety until they can be resolved. Additionally, MA results in diagnoses of DCIS for a subset of women and this leads to surgery and radiography of unproven value. Finally, the financial costs associated with MA are unacceptably high, an estimated $94 000 for every QALY. This is around double any reasonable cost limit and is therefore ethically unsupportable given the many less promoted but far more worthy needs that are starved of funds.

Why the question marks hanging over the true value of MA have not been obvious to the professions involved and (via the media) to the public is a matter of great concern. The *New York Times* editorial mentioned a strong possibility: the reluctance of the medical world to give up on what is an important source of income for many hospitals and doctors.[12] It is also significant that perhaps the most influential organization in this field, the American Cancer Society, has had five radiologists as former presidents.[15] Still another reason is that the cost-effectiveness calculations that have been done are based on the older, flawed trial data, and they incorporate some of the other biases mentioned in Chapter 1 and in Chapter 11.

Unfortunately, the medical establishment has become so powerful in the USA and in other Western countries that it can write its own ticket. And it has powerful allies as shown by the intervention by the US Congress and the White House when they promoted this medical procedure. But, it is vitally important to bear in mind that what is good (profitable, career-promoting) for the medical conglomerate has never been a trustworthy guideline for what is good for the public.

References

1   Brawley OW (2004) Prostate cancer screening: clinical applications and challenges. *Urol Oncol.* **22**: 353–7.
2   Frankel S, Smith GD, Donovan J and Neal D (2003) Screening for prostate cancer. *Lancet.* **361**: 1122–8.
3   Nyström L, Andersson I, Bjurstam N, Frisell J, Nordenskjöld B and Rutqvist LE (2002) Long-term effects of mammography screening: updated overview of the Swedish trials. *Lancet.* **359**: 909–19.
4   Humphrey LL, Helfand M, Benjamin KSC and Woolf SH (2002) Breast cancer screening: a summary of the evidence for the U.S. Preventive Services Task Force. *Ann Intern Med.* **137**: 347–60.
5   US Preventive Services Task Force (2002) Screening for breast cancer: Recommendations and rational. *Ann Intern Med.* **137**: 344–6.
6   Gøtzsche PC and Olsen O (2000) Is screening for breast cancer with mammography justifiable? *Lancet.* **355**: 129–34.
7   Olsen O and Gøtzsche PC (2001) Cochrane review on screening for breast cancer with mammography. *Lancet.* **358**: 1340–2.
8   Olsen O and Gøtzsche PC (2003) Screening for breast cancer with mammography (Cochrane Review). The Cochrane Library (1). Update Software, Oxford. Also available through *Lancet* (www.thelancet.com).
9   Baum M (2004) Commentary: false premises, false promises and false positives –the case against mammographic screening for breast cancer. *Int J Epidemiol.* **33**: 66–7.
10 Horton R (2001) Screening mammography – an overview revisited. *Lancet.* **358**: 1284–5.
11 Charatan F (2002) US panel finds insufficient evidence to support mammography. *BMJ.* **324**: 255.
12 Charatan F (2002) The great American mammography debate. *BMJ.* **324**: 432.
13 Foucar E (1996) Carcinoma-in-situ of the breast: have pathologists run amok? *Lancet.* **347**: 707–8.
14 Page DL and Jensen RA (1996) Ductal carcinoma in situ of the breast. *JAMA.* **275**: 948–9.
15 Epstein SS, Bertel R and Searman B (2001) Dangers and unreliability of mammography: breast examination is a safe, effective and practical alternative. *Int J Health Service.* **31**: 605–15.
16 Ernster VL, Ballard-Barbash, Barlow WE *et al.* (2002) Detection of ductal carcinoma in situ in women undergoing screening mammography. *J Natl Cancer Inst.* **94**: 1546–54.
17 Reeves K and Tatum C (2005) Columbus, OH: Ohio State University Medical Center; 2005. Available from http://jamesline.com/professionals/features.cfm?ID=1516 (accessed October 24, 2005).
18 Elmore JG, Barton MB, Moceri VM, Polk S, Arena PJ and Fletcher SW (1998) Ten-year risk of false positive screening mammograms and clinical breast examinations. *N Engl J Med.* **338**: 1089–96.
19 Public Health Agency of Canada (2005) Available from www.hc-sc.gc.ca (accessed November 4, 2005).
20 Arias E (2004) United States Life Tables, 2002. *National Vital Statistics Report 53.* Center for Disease Control. Available from www.cdc.gov/nchs/data/nvsr/nvsr53/nvsr53_06.pdf (accessed November 4, 2005).

Chapter 14

Screening for cervical cancer by Pap tests

Andrew Thompson and Norman J. Temple

Please note that an Appendix to this chapter can be found on the Radcliffe website (www.radcliffe-oxford.com/medicalspending).

Introduction

In this chapter we apply a critical eye to the subject of the Pap test for the prevention of cervical cancer (CC). The widely accepted wisdom is that thanks to this screening procedure deaths from CC in many countries are only about half of what they would be otherwise. Now who in their right mind would condemn thousands of women to a needless death from this cancer if it can be easily prevented? But, as we shall attempt to demonstrate, when we make a careful evaluation of the hard facts, what we find is that the Pap test is, in reality, an expensive way to extend lives. This is especially the case if the screening guidelines lead doctors to perform the test on too many women and with too great a frequency.

In many countries women are advised to be screened for CC by use of the Pap test every two to five years, starting around age 20 and continuing to at least age 65. This screening program has been well received, most notably in the USA but also in Canada, the UK, and other developed countries.[1]

The Pap test involves taking a smear of cells from the cervix, examining it for any lesions, and determining how advanced the lesions are. Like all forms of medical diagnosis, including all types of screening for cancer, the test is far from foolproof. Indeed, the whole process of screening and interpreting is complex and often leads to equivocal test results. First, we have false negatives. Because any lesion might be present in only a small fraction of the cervix, the sample might not contain any cells from an area with a lesion. Similarly, due to the difficulty of preparing and interpreting the samples, abnormal cells might be present but not be detected by the examiner.[2] The problem presented by false negatives is that an opportunity is lost to carry out a preventive intervention. With false positives, by contrast, alarm bells are set off by mistake and a woman is subjected to unnecessary repeat Pap tests, and perhaps precautionary removal of tissue up to and including total hysterectomy. The range of incorrect results was found, in a 1999 review, to range from zero to 30%. The reviewers could not be more certain since sufficient precautions to avoid bias were taken in only three of the 84 studies.[2]

The vital question we need to answer is as follows: When we add up all the costs of screening women using the Pap test, and then factor in problems that arise from false positives, is the benefit achieved by the reduction in deaths from CC really worth the resources expended?

Adverse effects from false positives

In order to gain insight into the problem of false positives, we first have to determine how many women undergo one or more investigative procedures? Our best information probably comes from a study which examined the cervical screening records of 350 000 British women, aged 20–64, from 1976 to 1996.[3] For every 10 000 women, 1564 of them had abnormal smears, leading to 818 investigations, and finding 514 with abnormal tissue. Yet, the expected rate of women who might be expected to develop invasive CC in any given year was never greater than three per 10 000, and lifetime risk is less than 1%.[4] This indicates that at least 27 abnormal results are found for each case of actual CC.

Another study also demonstrated the large amount of testing required as a result of false positives. This study was of 2561 postmenopausal women who had a normal test within the two previous years. The investigators then found 103 of them with mild to moderate abnormalities after the first year, but no "positive test result." After two years 110 abnormalities were found, one of which was diagnosed as positive, but none had high-grade lesions, much less invasive cancer. To reach these conclusions required almost 300 additional investigative procedures, including 33 colposcopies (in which the cervix is examined under magnification) and 21 biopsies.[5]

All of these investigative procedures have adverse side effects. However, determining the full extent of this is problematic as shown by a report of the screening of 226 000 women in the UK. This study found that about one in every 15 was told that there was a possible abnormality, but only one-third of them had actual treatment. However, all the women with a possible abnormality were "left with problems that include lasting worries about cancer, difficulties in obtaining life insurance, and worries concerning the effect of their treatment on their subsequent reproductive ability."[6]

A report of a study designed to find a means to improve on the accuracy of the Pap test describes some other consequences.[7]

> *Current management often includes colposcopy-directed biopsy to confirm the severity of the disease, and cervical ablation [removal by electrophysical means such as laser surgery] or excision of even low grade or equivocal lesions ... to prevent progression ... The cost of these services and subsequent overtreatment is considerable. Medical complications of treatment are rare, but include cervical incompetence, secondary infertility, infection, and cervical stenosis [narrowing of the cervical neck]. Furthermore, emotional concerns regarding referral and treatment for persistent viral infections and "precancerous conditions" are sometimes substantial.*

The authors note that most of the lesions will either regress spontaneously or are benign. However, out of concern that some more important lesions may be missed and out of fear of litigation arising from "unreasonable societal expectations of perfect cancer prevention," removal is done immediately of all suspect tissue rather than following up the findings at a later date.

It seems the screening campaign for Pap tests has led to expensive overprevention with potentially serious physical and psychological harm to some recipients.

Efficacy of screening by Pap tests

We now have an idea of the procedures that are associated with screening for CC using the Pap test and of its adverse effects due to the large numbers of false positives. We also know that almost all women "should" have the test regularly, and, indeed, that most women do so in well-off countries. But how effective are Pap tests at preventing CC and at what expense? Alas, the evidential base has never really been established that can provide accurate answers to these questions.

A 1990 article by Eddy[8] summarized the nature of the evidence up to that point. He called it "indirect evidence." It consists of "historical studies, case–control studies, analysis of data from large screening programs, and analysis of the natural history of cervical cancer with mathematical models." What is notably missing is clinical trial information, the bedrock that should be present before one invests in a multibillion dollar mass screening program.

Unfortunately, the picture has not changed in the last 16 years. What has changed is the number of historical studies that have found declines in both incidence and mortality of invasive CC after the introduction of large-scale screening programs in various cities and countries. This is epidemiological evidence collected over long periods of time. It is therefore prone to a host of confounding changes, such as changes in the criteria for diagnosis, collection, and preservation of data, improvements in treatment, and changes in lifestyle, hygiene, and sexual practices.

Eddy[8] also cites a number of case–control studies (i.e. comparisons of women with and without CC). The control subjects were matched primarily by age, but not by several other variables that could affect the reliability of the findings, such as social level, obesity, whether the woman had ever been pregnant, or sexual activity. This latter is a major factor in terms of the risk of transmission of the human papilloma virus (HPV) believed to be responsible for most, perhaps all, cases of CC. Angela Raffle,[9] who has provided much of the information on which this chapter is based, discusses other errors in case–control studies of CC. A notable one is that those who volunteer for screening are often more health-conscious than those who do not, and this likely biases the results in favor of screening. We see, therefore, that the evidence that purports to demonstrate the effectiveness of screening for CC is prone to multiple sources of error.

Why has there not been a randomized trial to determine the efficacy of screening using the Pap test for the prevention of death from CC? It would make good scientific sense to do so before implementing large-scale screening programs. Belief that such screening works, based on theory and historical trend evidence, probably played a large role in the early days. Then as so often happens in medicine other motives take over. These range from a genuine desire to protect patients from harm, combined with trust in the experts that there is good evidence for the procedure, to fear of being sued if the physician fails to advocate screening, to the realization for some that this would be a large money-making and career-boosting opportunity.

Cost-effectiveness of screening using the Pap test

A proper cost-effectiveness estimate cannot be made because, as noted above, the long-term trial data have never been gathered that would reveal how much it actually costs to prevent one death from CC by screening. Instead, estimates are based on projections of how many "precancerous" findings lead to one death. However, such projections can exaggerate the danger. Raffle et al.[10] demonstrated how the "cure" rate can be exaggerated 90% by assuming that all potentially cancerous lesions found by screening were as likely to proceed to cancer as were those found before screening was introduced.

However, we will assume that there is some efficacy to Pap test screening and attempt to estimate the true cost. Given the lack of trial data, we, too, have to make some assumptions. We will start with the one study that would seem to have a good claim on reliability, namely the large UK study referred to earlier. We will use it as the basis for estimating how many women must be screened and how many tests must be carried out in order to prevent one death from CC. This means we will assume the same 60% reduction in CC mortality that the UK study did, as this accords with US estimates that most of the 70% reduction in CC mortality in the USA during the past 50 years is due to Pap tests.[11,12] We will use American cost estimates for the Pap tests and other procedures involved.

The obvious ingredients of a cost estimate are the costs of the office visit, the taking and processing of the Pap test and of any repeat tests, of colposcopy to investigate suspect findings, of biopsy of suspect tissue, and of ablation or surgery. There are several other costs which should be included, such as organizing and sending invitations and reminders to women, computer systems for recording, performance monitoring, local and national coordination of the whole program, training and continuing education for the personnel involved, and publicizing and explaining the program.[13] Of course, some of these costs would inevitably accrue even without screening, notably as a result of women developing clinical symptoms of CC and then receiving treatment. Obtaining reliable estimates of all these costs of a screening program is extremely difficult, but listing them shows why any cost estimates are likely to be substantial underestimates. Out of necessity we will include only those costs which have been estimated, knowing they are far from being the full costs.

According to the UK study, 13 000 women, aged 24–64, would have to undergo screening every five years over a 20-year follow-up period to prevent or postpone one death from CC.[3] We adjusted these numbers based on screening guidelines from the American Cancer Society as they call for more frequent screening (every two or three years rather than every five years). Using these data, the estimated total cost for preventing one death from cervical cancer is about $10.7 million. (*See* the appendix on the website for details of the calculations.)

However, 20 years is an insufficient time to determine the full value of such preventive screening. Hence, it was decided to extend mathematically the study another 15 years (to 35 years). The effect of this projection is that the number of women who must be screened for one death from CC to be prevented falls from 13 000 to 1000.[3] Based on these figures the estimated total cost for preventing one death from cervical cancer is about $1.15 million.

To summarize so far, depending on the numbers used and the timespan involved, the total cost for preventing or postponing one death from CC is anywhere from about $1.15 million to $10.7 million.

In the next step we need to estimate the number of quality-adjusted life years (QALYs) that screening provides. To do this we must bear in mind that as no randomized, controlled long-term trial has been carried out, we really do not know how many years of extended life women gain on average when death from CC is prevented. In actuality, the number of years gained is likely to be significantly less than that of an average woman of the same age who never had CC. This is because several risk factors for CC, such as smoking and a low socioeconomic status,[14,15] are also closely associated with an increased risk of premature death from a host of other diseases. Given this it would be reasonable to assume that women whose deaths from CC are prevented have, on average, a lifespan that is somewhat shorter than that of other women. As detailed in the appendix on the website, we estimate that the cost per QALY is $711 000 or $95 800, based on 20 or 35 years of screening, respectively.

Conclusion

We have now looked at the cost for prevention of one death from CC in the USA. The costs are enormous: between $1.15 million and $10.7 million. This high cost is inevitable in view of the fact that invasive CC is a relatively uncommon disease: American women have less than one chance in 100 of developing it. These cost estimates, of course, have much imprecision. They are unlikely to include all the important costs that we listed previously, such as the costs for testing laboratories, recording and monitoring all the relevant data, and the training and continuing education of staff for the program. We really do not have an accurate answer to two key questions: How effective is the Pap test for reducing the risk of death from CC? and How many years of extra life are generated when death from CC is prevented?

Our estimates of the cost per QALY range from $95 800 and $711 000. These figures should be compared with our proposed cost limit per QALY, as stated in Chapter 1, of $50 000 as a medium-term goal and $27 000 as both an ideal limit and a longer-term goal. This indicates that the Pap test, as presently utilized in the USA, is a financially extravagant means to improve the health of the population. Quite apart from the financial cost, we need to reiterate that the gains to the tiny minority whose deaths from CC are prevented are counterbalanced by the psychological and physical harms to the far greater numbers who have treatment not destined to save their lives.

The cost-effectiveness of screening varies considerably based on how it is used. The estimations made here were based on the American Cancer Society guidelines, which call for a Pap test every two or three years. However, Raffle[16] argued for far fewer tests. Her proposal was to use the test only for women between the ages of 25 and 50, and with tests carried out every five years, not every three years (she was discussing proposed changes to British screening guidelines). If these suggestions were implemented, this would hugely improve the cost-effectiveness of screening. A focus on women at high risk would also go far to achieving this vital goal. In particular, as women who have had multiple sexual partners are most likely to contract the HPV virus that is thought to cause most, if not all, cases, then screening should be more concentrated on these women, or those who are positive for the virus.

Screening for CC may therefore resemble the use of statins: yes, the medical intervention does postpone deaths, and yes, the more it is used, the more deaths that are postponed. But when the people who write the guidelines become over-zealous in their determination to maximize the number of lives "saved," the procedure quickly becomes one more case of a Rolls Royce medicine. Clearly, more research is required to determine what guidelines are most appropriate.

Screening for CC, as currently practiced, harms the public. First, it diverts funds from more effective disease-prevention interventions. And, second, it subjects thousands of women to psychological and physical harm that arises from the unnecessary procedures that result from this testing. One wonders at the objectivity of most of the designated experts in this field. For example, of the seven authors of the current guidelines of the American Cancer Society, all but one reported having multiple financial ties to commercial enterprises.[11]

It is hoped that a new screening methodology will be developed which is more accurate and less expensive. Before acceptance, it should undergo examination by randomized controlled trials and cost-effectiveness analyses, perhaps first by using it on those who are at especially high risk of developing CC.

Acknowledgment

We are grateful to Dr Angela Raffle for valuable information.

References

1 Grady D (2002) Fewer Pap tests advised for some by U.S. group. *New York Times*, December 19: 6.
2 Nuovo J, Melnikow J and Howell LP (2001) New tests for cervical cancer screening. *Am Fam Physician*. **64**: 729–30.
3 Raffle AE, Alden B, Quinn M, Babb PJ and Brett MT (2003) Outcomes of screening to prevent cancer: analysis of cumulative incidence of cervical abnormality and modelling of cases and deaths prevented. *BMJ*. **326**: 901–10.
4 Raffle AE (1998) New tests in cervical screening. *Lancet*. **351**: 297.
5 Sawaya GF, Grady D, Kerlikowske K *et al.* (2000) The positive predictive value of cervical smears in previously screened postmenopausal women: the heart and estrogen/progestin replacement study (HERS). *Ann Intern Med*. **133**: 942–50.
6 Raffle AE (1999) How long will screening myths survive. *Lancet*. **354**: 431.
7 Schiffman M and Adrianza ME (2000) ASCUS-LSIL triage study. *Acta Cytology*. **44**: 726–42.
8 Eddy DE (1990) Screening for cervical cancer. *Ann Intern Med*. **113**: 214–6.
9 Raffle AE (2003) Commentary: case–control studies of screening should carry a health warning. *Int J Epidemiol*. **32**: 577–8.
10 Raffle AE, Alden B and Mackenzie EFD (1999) Detection rates for abnormal cervical smears: what are we screening for? *Lancet*. **345**: 1469–73.
11 Saslow D, Runowicz CD, Solomon D *et al.* (2002) American Cancer Society Guideline for the early detection of cervical neoplasia and cancer. *CA Cancer J Clin*. **52**: 342–62.
12 Minnesota Department of Health (1999) *New Technologies for Cervical Cancer Screening*. January. Available from www.health.state.mm.us/htac/Pap.htm (accessed September 15, 2004).
13 Raffle AE (2002) *Programme Map for Cervical Screening*. October. Sent by A Raffle, September 9, 2004. (Unpublished.)

14 Trimble CL, Genkinger JM, Burke AE *et al.* (2005) Active and passive cigarette smoking and the risk of cervical neoplasia. *Obstet Gynecol.* **105**: 174–81.

15 McFadden K, McConnell D, Salmond C, Crampton P and Fraser J (2004) Socioeconomic deprivation and the incidence of cervical cancer in New Zealand: 1988–1998. *NZ Med J.* **117**: U1172.

16 Raffle AE (2004) Cervical screening. *BMJ.* **328**: 1272–3.

Note by the editors

Up to this point in the book we have being painting a picture of the problems apparent in so much of the medical enterprise, including the pharmaceutical industry, with an emphasis on financial waste. But in the final four chapters we use a different telescope, the one without the crosshairs. From here the focus is no longer "this is how things are being done wrongly," but rather "this is how things could and should be done."

Chapter 15

Paying for what works: the Reference Drug Program as a model for rational policy-making

Alan Cassels and Norman J. Temple

Introduction

In the Canadian province of British Columbia (BC) the provincial government implemented a policy that was designed to restrain drug costs. This policy is of much interest, both for its own sake and also as a lesson as to how the drug industry proactively responds to perceived threats to its profits.

The BC Pharmacare program is the publicly funded drug insurance program operated by the BC Ministry of Health. In the early 1990s its budget was rising rapidly. In 1995, in response to this problem, Pharmacare introduced the Reference Drug Program (RDP), initially called "Reference-based pricing." This policy grew out of a number of other cost-containment policies.

RDP is an example of policy-makers attempting to apply an evidence-based approach to decisions on drug coverage. In many ways implementing RDP in BC set a bold new paradigm in terms of controlling public drug expenditures in Canada. The rationale behind RDP is simple: if there is no evidence that a newer, more expensive drug is therapeutically superior to a cheaper treatment, the program should fund the least expensive alternative first. If, for whatever reason, the cheaper drug does not work for a particular patient, the physician can apply to have a more expensive medication covered or the patient can choose to pay the extra cost. Although the policy possesses a simple commonsense appeal, its introduction led to much controversy.

A more common strategy in Canada were policies that, according to the Canadian Institute of Health Information (CIHI), saw public officials react to increasing drug costs by shifting costs to consumers with higher user fees or premiums. When added costs get shifted to consumers or private insurance plans, the manufacturers are less likely to be directly affected than if the government starts implementing value-for-money assessments of new drugs. With RDP, and other policies which reject paying for specific products because they do not have therapeutic advantages over older or cheaper products, the BC government witnessed the manufacturers mobilize political lobbying, advertising, and public relations capabilities in an effort to kill such a policy.

By 1995, various forms of reference pricing were in place in the Netherlands, Denmark, and New Zealand, while Italy had announced plans to implement such a policy. Each country used a different approach and succeeded in producing price reductions.[1-3] The pharmaceutical industry argued on a number of grounds that the policies in those countries were failures, but convincing evidence to support such claims has never been presented. These reports often describe failure as the inability of RDP programs to contain costs at or near the rate of inflation.Any drug policy, such as RDP, that restricts formulary access based on price will be controversial because it attacks the modern pharmaceutical industry's emphasis on innovation – that unique differences in chemicals merit unique differences (usually premiums) in price. In order for the drug industry to expand and return growing profits to shareholders, drug differences have to be found or created, and then exploited.

Clearly, governments which are highly selective about which drugs to reimburse inevitably clash with a core strategy of the pharmaceutical manufacturers: profit maximization by creating and marketing easier-to-produce "me-too" patented formulations and then charging the maximum that the market will bear. This point was clearly shown in Chapter 6. The agency in Canada charged with countering this is the Patented Medicines Prices Review Board (PMPRB). It allows prices of new drugs that offer, at most, a moderate therapeutic improvement to be priced to the maximum of other drugs in their class, but not beyond. The PMPRB may prevent some excessive pricing of new drugs in Canada but many argue that Canadians are still paying too much for drugs due to the guaranteed 20-year patent monopoly they are afforded.

Pharmaceutical companies typically invest much more on marketing their products than they do on creating and studying the chemical entity in the first place. US Public Citizen, a health watchdog group based in Washington, DC, found that in 2000, the 11 Fortune 500 drug companies devoted 30% of their revenue to marketing and administrative costs but only 12% to research and development.[4] These numbers allow us to safely conclude that exaggeration of even the subtlest interpretations of therapeutic advantage brings a higher return than actually producing innovation in the first place. The marketing tactics of the pharmaceutical industry were discussed in Chapter 5.

If a new drug does not hold up to independent scientific examination and is thought to be no better or no more cost-effective than existing treatments, it follows that only an irrational or misled person would pay a premium price for it. The sad truth is that most new drugs, when examined independently, do not provide any additional therapeutic benefit compared to drugs already in the market. In a recent analysis of new drugs approved in the USA between 1982 and 1991, more than half (53%) had "little or no therapeutic gain" compared to drugs already in the market, and only 16% of new drugs represented an "important therapeutic gain."[4]

Background: the cost pressures on BC Pharmacare

Like most drug benefits plans in the industrialized world, BC Pharmacare has to contend with serious and mounting cost pressures. In the early 1990s the cost of this program was increasing at a rate of 16% per year. Canada's overall drug expenditure grew an average of 12.1% per year from 1985 to 1992.[5] As a result the share of total healthcare spending allocated to drugs grew from 8.4% in the late 1970s to 14.5% in 1997. According to the CIHI, in 1997, for the first time since comparable detailed expenditure data had been compiled (1975), spending on drugs became the second-largest category of total health expenditure, overtaking spending on physician services. By 2002 more than 16% of all healthcare spending was for drugs.[6]

The drivers behind cost rises in drug coverage have been extensively analyzed.[7] Some of the main factors are the costs per prescription, number of prescriptions, the number of plan beneficiaries, and the population size. The leading factor responsible for overall growth was the number of prescriptions dispensed, which increased by 47% between 1990 and 1998. The next factor was the average cost per prescription, which increased by 34%. The number of beneficiaries and the growing population contributed 42% and 22%, respectively, to this growth in spending. In 1993, an independent research paper examined the reasons for the Pharmacare growing budget and concluded that 34% of the cost increase was due to costlier new drugs or increased prices of old drugs.[8] The paper also concluded that population aging had almost nothing to do with increased drug use. The fact that newer, more expensive products were replacing older, cheaper drugs should encourage any drug benefits policy planner to adopt a general strategy of avoiding higher priced, newer drugs that are essentially therapeutic duplicates of existing drugs.

There are other factors that might also help explain this cost growth. Reform of the healthcare system continues to emphasize alternatives to institutionalization. For that reason more pharmaceuticals are being developed and applied to a wider variety of conditions and diseases with the aim of keeping people out of hospitals. To the degree that pharmaceuticals are deemed to be safe and effective alternatives to institutionalization, this upward pressure on the volume of drugs consumed can be expected to intensify.

RDP and other cost-containment policies

The RDP should be seen as part of a variety of cost-containment policies which have been enacted in BC. It is seen by some as a logical extension of the Low Cost Alternative Program (LCA), a policy also known as "generic substitution," which mandates Pharmacare to pay for the least expensive alternative when chemically identical drugs are supplied by different companies. The goal of both RDP and LCA was to provide similar coverage for similar drugs without increasing other health service costs or adverse health events.

Other mechanisms have been implemented by Pharmacare to help control drug plan costs. These include the following.

- Reducing the maximum supply for short-term therapy drugs from 100 days to 30 days. This reduces waste from unused larger prescription size.
- Expanding the range of drugs affected by the trial prescription program. Under this program costlier medications are targeted for initial fills as trial prescriptions (14 days' supply). A national analysis of trial prescription programs showed that they are acceptable to patients and, if focused on specific medications, can reduce the costs associated with drug wastage.[9]
- Auditing PharmaNet transactions for fraud and abuse. This involves identifying patients or pharmacies suspected of fraud, investigating them, and working to recover costs.

- Restricted Claimants Program reduces abusive prescription drug behavior among extremely high users who may be selling drugs or otherwise taking excessive amounts.
- PharmaNet, the province-wide pharmacy computer network implemented in 1995, helped to lower administrative costs and deliver faster adjudication of claims. This system expedites the Special Authority program which encourages cost-effective prescribing while ensuring access to necessary care. Current administrative costs are around 1% of Pharmacare's overall budget.

Despite relatively good drug coverage for seniors and those on social assistance in most provinces, even small changes in co-payments or deductibles can influence individual access to necessary drugs. As a result, when jurisdictions try to shift growing costs to consumers or private-sector insurance plans, they sometimes set up a system that sacrifices equity (where the poorest tend to suffer the most) for cost savings. Reducing access to "essential drugs," such as insulin and anti-arrhythmia agents, can increase hospitalizations and deaths. Because of this, many other jurisdictions, in particular in Europe, prefer to try more equitable alternatives to expanding patient cost-sharing schemes. Some jurisdictions use co-payment schemes that would appear to have little impact on the poor. The UK, for instance, has steadily increased co-payments while continuing to exempt about 80% of people receiving prescription drugs. Because RDP did not affect the level of co-payments or deductibles facing consumers, the policy had no effect on access to essential medicines.

Any drug benefits policy that has a restricted list of drugs it is willing to pay for must rely on an unbiased and scientifically valid assessment of the added benefits of new drugs. If those benefits are not seen to justify additional expenditures, it follows that consumers, private drug plans, or public drug insurance plans would be acting irrationally if they opted to pay for the more expensive – but not more effective – drugs. The point was well put by Maclure and colleagues[10] in one of the most exhaustive papers on RDP in BC: "If there is no evidence that a higher price buys better effectiveness or fewer toxicities, then the extra cost should not be covered in a publicly funded insurance program."

The Therapeutics Initiative (TI) was created in 1994, with funding from the BC Ministry of Health, in order to create an independent source of scientific expertise. This group of clinicians and pharmacists at the University of British Columbia reviews published evidence of the clinical effectiveness of new drugs and provides its evaluations to BC health professionals and to Pharmacare and its Drug Benefit Committee. The latter committee is the sole authority for making decisions on drug listings.

If patients meet certain criteria that indicate an adverse effect from a switch in medications, or if they are intolerant to the reference drug, they can be exempted from the policy if physicians submit an appropriate form. In some cases, if the prescriber is a specialist, he or she may be authorized to make exemptions to the policy. If patients wish to take a more expensive drug and have not been exempted from the policy, they can choose to pay the extra cost.

What was referenced in the RDP?

The RDP was applied to five classes of drugs between October 1995 and January 1997. It has not been extended to other classes.

H_2-antagonists

The histamine-2 receptor antagonists are used in the treatment of non-ulcer dyspepsia or upper gastrointestinal tract complaints. The TI reviewed these drugs in 1994 and found that that there was little difference between the various agents other than cost.[11] It was estimated that costs of daily use of cimetidine ($0.14 per day) is only one-third the cost of the next most expensive H_2-antagonist, ranitidine ($0.44 per day).

Nitrates

Used in the treatment of angina. The BC Office of Health Technology Assessment found no evidence of significant differences between regular release isosorbide dinitrate (ISDN) and oral nitroglycerine (SR-NG).[12] The most significant difference between the two was the 10-fold higher cost of SR-NG.

NSAIDs

Nonsteroidal anti-inflammatory drugs (NSAIDs) are used in the treatment of osteoarthritis and rheumatism. The class of NSAIDs consists of many therapeutically equivalent products with large differences in price. No specific NSAID has been shown to have superior efficacy or lower overall toxicity. Experience with a prior authorization program for NSAIDs as part of Medicaid in Tennessee enabled managers to reduce NSAID expenditures by 53% during the following two years for an estimated savings of $12.8 million.[13] The reduction in expenditures resulted from the increased use of generic NSAIDs, as well as from a 19% decrease in overall NSAID use.

The TI review of February 1995 identified relatively few clinical trials comparing the effectiveness of different NSAIDs. These trials have not demonstrated any consistent superiority of one NSAID over another.[14] Differences reported in publications can often be explained by the fact that the studies did not use equivalent doses.[15]

ACE inhibitors

Angiotensin-converting enzyme (ACE) inhibitors are used in the treatment of hypertension. Any ACE inhibitor will control blood pressure in 50% to 70% of patients. There are few clinically significant differences between ACE inhibitors.[16]

CCBs

Calcium channel blockers (CCBs) are another class of drugs used in the treatment of hypertension. Any one CCB will effectively control blood pressure in 60% to 70% of patients. Only dihydropyridines are included under the RDP.

Evaluating RDP: controlling for confounding factors and establishing the evidence base

When the costs but not the effectiveness of drugs within a class vary substantially, limiting reimbursement to the cost of the lowest-priced drug will likely reduce prescription drug expenditures. However, there is a chance that the pricing policy could inadvertently increase overall healthcare costs if the referenced drugs are not actually interchangeable in terms of benefit and risk. A series of independent analyses of the five categories of drugs that were referenced in BC showed ''little evidence to indicate that referenced drugs are not therapeutically equivalent within each of the drug classes.''[16]

The best study design in any policy evaluation would look at key indicators, such as the policy's impact on healthcare utilization or hospitalizations before and after RDP, while controlling extensively for other factors which could confound the findings (e.g. other changes in the health system, other concomitant drug policy changes, physician strikes, new drugs entering the market, and changes at the political level). Such care in designing and carrying out the study is necessary in order to determine the credibility of claims that RDP was responsible for increased rates of medical services use and hospitalizations.

Fortunately for BC, the ability to access PharmaNet and hospital data for evaluative purposes, coupled with a high level of methodological rigor demanded of the evaluations, attracted some of the best drug policy researchers in Canada and the USA to participate in evaluations. With funding from the BC Ministry of Health and other federal Canadian and American sources, independent researchers from several universities were involved in evaluating different aspects of RDP; these researchers were from the University of Victoria,[17,18] Harvard University,[19] McMaster University,[16] the University of Washington,[20] and the University of British Columbia.[21]

Impact on healthcare utlization and hospitalizations

Overall, the evaluations of RDP in BC have indicated that the policy has had no detectable adverse impact on healthcare utilization. McGregor[22] reported in the *Canadian Journal of Cardiology*: ''There has been no increase in physicians' office visits or in the rates of hospitalization of seniors associated with any of the sentinel illnesses [since the introduction of RDP in 1995].''

The policy's individual evaluations and findings are broken down by drug category as follows.

H_2-antagonists

The Pharmaceutical Outcomes Research and Policy Program at the University of Washington, Seattle, under Thomas Hazlet, analyzed the impact of RDP on H_2-antagonists. His analysis shows the policy "caused no increases in offices visits, ER visits, or hospitalizations."[20]

Nitrates

Paul Grootendorst and Anne Holbrook at the Centre for Evaluation of Medicines at McMaster University, Hamilton, Canada, studied the impact of the nitrate policy. Analyses confirmed that RDP saved more than $3 million per year and there was no increase in spending on beta-blockers or CCBs.[23]

Antihypertensives

Steven Soumerai and Sebastian Schneeweiss of Harvard University examined the impact of RDP on drug switching with ACE inhibitors. They found that the policy saved $6.7 million in the first 12 months, although many patients did not stop taking the more expensive non-reference ACE inhibitor. Schneeweiss presented results at a scientific conference in 2001 and reported that RDP for ACE inhibitors "appears to have successfully reduced pharmacological expenditures without an increase in use of the healthcare system."[24]

Opposition to the RDP: PMAC, physicians, and the Fraser Institute

Opposition to the RDP from the Pharmaceutical Manufacturers Association of Canada (PMAC, which is now called Rx&D) was swift and pre-emptive. PMAC, which represented the brand name drug industry in Canada, initiated a series of full-page advertisements in major BC newspapers months before the policy was implemented in an attempt to generate public opposition and discredit the policy. Opposition also came from other provincial health professional and consumer organizations that had little in common except their willingness to lobby against the RDP policy and perhaps their disagreement with the governing party.

If any drug policy creates more work for harried physicians and pharmacists without appropriate compensation, opposition to that policy can be expected. RDP did not win many friends among pharmacists. While it did pay pharmacists for their extra time in some cases, there was a perceived lack of consultation on rolling out the policy. On top of this, the timing created problems as it arrived at about the same time as the BC pharmacy network system, PharmaNet.

One of the main criticisms of RDP was the alleged involvement of the ministry in prescribing decisions. The Canadian Cardiovascular Society delivered a position paper in 1996 criticizing RDP by saying that physicians were being second-guessed by ministry bureaucrats. RDP's escape clause was the "special authority process" whereby physicians could fax a request to Pharmacare to obtain coverage for their patients who they felt needed a more expensive drug than the reference one. It is possible that physicians resented the added paperwork for which they were not compensated, and it is not surprising that many physicians saw RDP as an infringement on their prescribing.[25] The main criticism was not the perception of bureaucratic influence on prescribing but that physicians felt they were not adequately consulted in the creation or implementation of the policy. In one qualitative study of RDP, the attitudes of physicians, pharmacists, and seniors towards the policy were studied in focus groups. Researchers found that clinicians "felt that the policy had been imposed on them without consultation, creating a situation whereby they must promote a policy in which they had no say and have no confidence."[18]

The Fraser Institute, a conservative think-tank, summed up its corporate-backed opposition to the policy by penning a paper calling RDP a "dangerous and costly mistake." The author, Bill McArthur, said that: "Reference pricing has been implemented in other countries, and repeatedly it has exhibited two fundamental flaws, one medical and the other economic. From a medical viewpoint it is associated with increased illness. From an economic standpoint it increases healthcare costs substantially."[26] However, McArthur relied on mostly ideologically based assertions and not evidence to substantiate these points.

The rhetorical war over RDP

The governing party in BC at the time was the left-of-center New Democratic Party (NDP). The NDP government saw itself as displaying immense courage by acting as the guardian of the public purse by implementing a policy that prevents excessive profits by the pharmaceutical industry. PMAC countered that the government was fiddling in the public's medicine cabinet, a place it clearly did not belong. In fact, the battle over RDP was dominated by a great deal of entertaining and fiery rhetoric on both sides. PMAC proclaimed in full-page newspaper adverts, "The Provincial Government wants to change your medication." The provincial government countered with equal invective. One newspaper headline proclaimed: "Minister condemns drug manufacturers. Greedy multinational firms trying to terrorize British Columbians".[27] At least in the ensuing verbal jousting and political posturing the provincial NDP found fresh reasons to distrust the drug industry and the drug industry was given new ammunition to oppose the governing NDP.

The opinions of average citizens were studied as part of research evaluating the impact of RDP on seniors. The study looked at the media messages used by the government and the drug industry and concluded that the fiscal merits of RDP seemed more credible with the public than the drug industry's rhetoric. In fact, studying consumer opinion revealed that the drug manufacturers' tactics generated a high degree of scepticism about their anti-RDP message. The authors concluded that the pharmaceutical industry's campaign was generally unsuccessful because "Pharmacare's messages resonated more effectively with seniors' views on public health policy."[17]

If they could not win in the court of public opinion, PMAC decided to try their luck in another court. In December 1995, PMAC and seven of its member companies filed a suit in the Supreme Court of BC to stop the Minister of Health and Pharmacare from implementing RDP. The courts ruled in the government's favor. Finally, in February 1998, the Supreme Court of Canada refused to hear the case. Despite this legal defeat, PMAC's actions might have been a factor in dissuading the government from expanding RDP to other drug categories. How-ever, the real reason for this is not known.

Evaluation of the RDP

Although critics of the policy claimed that RDP was never properly evaluated, the degree to which Pharmacare encouraged independent evaluation of its policy set an impressive precedent for the BC health system. Results from a 1998 provincial audit of Pharmacare included, as one of 10 recommendations, the suggestion that Pharmacare should encourage independent reviews of RDP and report the results to key stakeholders.[28] Strong demands for evaluation also came from physicians' organizations and the drug industry, which were interested in any evidence to support their viewpoint that the policy was a failure. The clamoring has been an unexpected boon for the program as it has made RDP in BC probably the most thoroughly evaluated drug policy in the history of the Canadian drug benefit plans.

As with most research, initial findings largely concluded that more study is needed. For example, a PMAC-funded study in 1999 concluded that despite initial and dramatic declines in annual expenditures due to RDP, "a more comprehensive and longitudinal evaluation of reference-based pricing is needed and should take into account a wide range of non-cost impacts, the most important of which are the effects on health outcomes."[29] Fortunately, decision-makers within the BC Ministry of Health invested money into attracting outside researchers to lead evaluations of RDP, which could be done with rigor and precision.

There are two main financial effects that could have been caused by an RDP policy change. The first and most obvious is the impact on the Pharmacare budget. If the policy saves money, either by reducing the rate of increase or keeping program spending static, it could be deemed at least partly successful. The second is that the policy must demonstrate that it is maintaining equivalent coverage of appropriate medicine without increasing other health costs, such as doctor visits and hospitalizations. The ability of researchers to link PharmaNet data with hospital and Medical Services Plan data meant that the impact of the policy could be carefully monitored.[30]

The Ministry of Health's own documents indicate the policy likely saved the province about $44 million in 1999.[31] Outside assessments done by independent researchers were able to verify some of the plan savings (notably with ACE inhibitors). None of the other evaluations revealed any evidence that RDP was responsible for overall increases or shifts of costs to other parts of the health system.

An early study on the experience of RDP confirmed that there were "dramatic declines in annual expenditures for drugs within referenced categories (from $42 million the year before reference-based pricing was introduced to $23.7 million the year after)." The authors suggested that this study of RDP was preliminary and what was needed was a longer, comprehensive evaluation to examine its potential for non-cost effects such as health outcomes.[29]

One analysis of RDP, a commentary appearing in the May 2001 issue of the *Fraser Forum*, claimed that since RDP started, public spending on drugs in BC has dramatically increased compared with the rest of Canada.[32] This report is flawed in that it wrongly assumes that public spending in the rest of Canada did not contract relative to that in BC. This was attributed to cost-shifting policies in other provinces which the author failed to account for. Other Canadian provinces, such as Quebec, downloaded costs to consumers. A change in drug policy in Quebec introduced co-payments in the mid-1990s, shifting about $400 million of additional drug costs to individuals.

Critics of RDP claim that it did not work and that it did not save the amounts of money the government said it would. However, over the last 10 years in BC, the only years in which the rate of growth of Pharmacare has slackened or remained steady are 1994–1996 when LCA and RDP were implemented. By 1997, we see the rate of budget escalations resuming its pre-1994 slope.

Some of the attacks of reference pricing are based on weak evidence or are largely critical commentaries written by industry-funded experts. One study indicated that there were possible complications from switching patients to different ACE inhibitors.[33] However, this study was flawed and likely committed channelling bias (i.e. patients initially prescribed captopril were actually sicker than those prescribed enalapril or lisinopril). Similarly, there were claims from the New Zealand experience that asking patients to switch from one cholesterol-lowering drug to another led to an increase in cardiovascular deaths. However, the evidence for this is weak as the authors concluded that underdosing may have been a factor in this study and that this happened independently of the introduction of RDP.[34]

Other criticisms of RDP indicate the policy would have a very marginal impact on plan spending, but such criticisms are largely based on short-term analyses. In refutation of the view, some analysts found through economic modeling that reference pricing "exerted increased pressure on the suppliers of innovative drugs, causing them to lower their price to the [reference price] level almost without exception."[35] Similarly, the price of the more expensive nitrates in BC came down after RDP, a clear indication that some increased price competition would force manufacturers to lower their prices to the reference level.

It is true that cost savings, wherever reference pricing has been tried, have been variable. In Germany, where the policy was introduced in 1989, anticipated savings were not realized, largely because there was little difference in the cost among the generic products selected.[36] Others have stated that the German experience with RDP has been very good and has introduced price competition. Between 1991 and 1992 pharmaceutical firms decreased the prices of products affected by the reference system by 1.5%, whereas the prices of other drugs increased by 4.1%.[37] Evidence of program savings also comes from RDP's experience in other jurisdictions. In 1993 RDP was introduced in New Zealand. Before this, the drug expenditure budget was growing at a rate of 10% to 12% per year. To date, the New Zealand reference drug pricing program and other cost-saving measures have achieved cumulative savings of around US$185 million. Most noteworthy is that New Zealand's drug expenditure growth has slowed to 5.6% per year. The program has been expanded to include more therapeutic categories.

Conclusions and future policy options

It should be stressed that even if fully implemented, RDP is no panacea for slowing escalations of drug budgets. RDP is only one of many methods for controlling public drug expenditures. Other forms of cost control include use of generics, delistings, price negotiations, freezes, and limits on mark-up. RDP was seen to be most effective in price control in the few years after it was implemented. While total drug spending in the country continues to rise, even in the face of programs such as the RDP, governments need to recognize that, done properly and evaluated continuously, robust referencing systems are an important part of cost containment. Over time, the policy's effect seems to diminish, the causes of which are beyond the scope of this chapter.

According to the BC Ministry of Health, "The RDP program was developed to make Pharmacare more cost-effective and does not jeopardize a patient's health."[38] It is undeniable that the best evaluations have supported this claim. Nevertheless, it takes very strong government commitment to introduce a policy unfavorable to the interests of the pharmaceutical industry and then stand up to the considerable power of that industry. For whatever reason, whether it was pressure from professional groups, the government's preoccupation with other issues, or unspoken agreements with industry not to expand RDP (other than the nebulizer conversion policy in 1999), RDP expansion essentially froze in 1997. This is despite the fact that there are a number of drug categories where attractive savings could be achieved.

An appropriate test of whether an RDP program is succeeding is that it should have both a financial standard and a clinical standard; that is, it should reduce the growth rate of drug spending and neither transfer costs to other health sectors nor make patients worse off. Has RDP achieved these goals? One indication that it has done so is that in 2001 there were over a dozen countries employing some form of referencing of drug prices or are employing policies that only pay for the least expensive version of a drug.

Finally, it is worth mentioning again the experience of New Zealand, a nation demographically similar to BC. Their national drug subsidization program, PHARMAC, probably leads the world in its ability to contain drug costs through reference-based pricing, competitive bidding, and negotiating better prices with manufacturers. Although every drug benefits plan in the world is struggling with near double-digit cost growth, PHARMAC kept New Zealand's pharmaceutical expenditure growth to less than 6%. This is a remarkable feat, especially in light of the fact that such savings were achieved while also increasing the population's access to drugs. As the PHARMAC 2001 Annual Report noted "[PHARMAC] managed to provide access to a number of uniquely new chemical entities ... and that virtually all of these new listings were associated with targeting criteria."[39] Savings incurred by rigid drug plan cost control strategies means that other areas of the health system – hospital and home care – can be properly funded. Getting the right drug, to the right patient, at the lowest cost: now that is a paradigm for drug policy reform.

References

1 Selke G (1994) Reference price systems in the European Community. In: Mossialos E, Ranos C and Abel-Smith B, eds. *Cost Containment, Pricing and Financing of Pharmaceuticals in the European Community: the policy makers' view*. LSE Health and Pharmetrica SA, Athens.

2 New Zealand PHARMAC (1999) *Operating Policy and Procedures*. Available from www.pharmac.govt.nz/about/policy.html.

3 Jacobzone S (2000) *Pharmaceutical Policies in OECD Countries: reconciling social and industrial goals. Labour market and social policy*. Occasional Papers no. 40. Organisation for Economic

Co-operation and Development, Paris. Available from www.olis.oecd.org/OLIS/2000/DOC.NSF/LINKTO/DEELSA-ELSA-WD(2000)1.

4   Young B and Surrusco M (2001) Rx R&D myths: the case against the drug industry's R&D "scare card". *US Public Citizen Congress Watch.* 20.

5   CIHI (2002) *Drug Expenditures in Canada: 1985–2001.* Canadian Institutes of Health Information, Ottowa.

6   CIHI (2005) *Drug Expenditure in Canada: 1985–2004.* Canadian Institute for Health Information, Ottowa.

7   PMPRB (2002) *Provincial Drug Plans Overview Report: pharmaceutical trends 1995/96–1999/00.* Patent Medicines Prices Review Board, Ottowa.

8   Anderson GM, Kerluke KJ, Pulcins IR, Hertzman C and Barer ML (1993) Trends and determinants of prescription drug expenditures in the elderly: data from the British Columbia Pharmacare Program. *Inquiry.* **30:** 199–207.

9   Paterson JM and Anderson GM (2002) "Trial" prescriptions to reduce drug wastage: results from Canadian programs and a community demonstration project. *Am J Manag Care.* **8:** 151–8.

10 Maclure M, Nakagawa RS and Carleton BC (2001) *Applying Research to the Policy Cycle: implementing and evaluating evidence-based drug policies in British Columbia.* Milbank Quarterly series "Informing Judgment: case studies of health policy and research in six countries." Available from www.milbank.org/2001cochrane/010903cochrane.html#update.

11 Therapeutics Initiative (1994) *Newsletter,* 1. Available from www.ti.ubc.ca/pages/letter1.html.

12 Bassett K and Rhone M (1994) The efficacy and effectiveness of sustained release oral nitroglycerine in comparison to regular delivery isosorbide dinitrate for the prophylactic treatment of stable angina pectoris. BC Office of Health Technology Assessment: 1T.

13 Agency for Health Care Policy and Research (1997) *Meeting Medicaid's Cost and Quality Challenges: the role of AHCPR research.* AHCPR Program Note, AHCPR Publication No. 97–0044. AHCPR, Rockville, MD. Available from www.ahrq.gov/research/mednote.htm.

14 Therapeutics Initiative (1995) *Newsletter,* 4, February. Available from www.ti.ubc.ca/pages/letter4.html.

15 Rochon PA, Gurwitz JH, Simms RW *et al.* (1994) A study of manufacturer-supported trials of nonsteroidal anti-inflammatory drugs in the treatment of arthritis. *Arch Intern Med.* **154:** 157–63.

16 Grootendorst P and Holbrook A (1999) Evaluating the impact of reference-based pricing. *Can Med Assoc J.* **161:** 273–4.

17 Brunt JH, Chappell NL, Maclure M and Cassels A (1998) Assessing the effectiveness of government and industry media campaigns on seniors' perceptions of reference-based pricing policy. *J Applied Gerontology.* **17:** 276–95.

18 Mullett J and Coughlan R (1998) Clinicians' and seniors' views of reference based pricing: two sides of a coin. *J Applied Gerontology.* **17:** 296–317.

19 Schneeweiss S, Soumerai SB, Glynn RJ, Maclure M, Dormuth C and Walker AM (2002) Impact of reference-based pricing for angiotensin-converting enzyme inhibitors on drug utilization. *Can Med Assoc J.* **166:** 737–45.

20 Hazlet TK and Blough DK (2002) Health services utilization with reference drug pricing of histamine(2) receptor antagonists in British Columbia elderly. *Med Care.* **40:** 640–9.

21 Nakagawa B and Hudson R (2000) Reference-based pricing. *Can Med Assoc J.* **162:** 12, 14.

22 McGregor M (1998) Coverage of drug costs: reference-based pricing. *Can J Cardiology.* **14:** 666–8.

23 Grootendorst P, Dolovich L, O'Brien B, Holbrook A and Levy A (2001) Impact of reference-based pricing of nitrates on the use and costs of anti-anginal drugs. *Can Med Assoc J.* **165:** 1011–9.

24 Reuters News Agency (2001) *Reference-based drug pricing is effective, researchers find.* Report on the International Conference on Pharmacoepidemiology, August 31.

25 Woollard RF (1996) Opportunity lost: a frontline view of reference-based pricing. *Can Med Assoc J.* **154:** 1185–8.

26 McArthur W (1997) Reference-based pricing – a dangerous and costly mistake. *Fraser Forum,* January: 24–5.

27 Munro M (1995) Minister condemns drug manufacturers: greedy multinational firms trying to 'terrorize British Columbians'. *Vancouver Sun,* June 21: A3.

28 Morfitt G, Auditor General of BC Press Release (1998) *Pharmacare Controls Costs, Could Do More to Foster Appropriate Drug Use, says Auditor General*. Victoria: Province of British Columbia, August 11.

29 Narine L, Senathirajah M and Smith T (1999) Evaluating reference-based pricing: initial findings and prospects. *Can Med Assoc J*. **161**: 286–8.

30 Bellet G (2001) BC government attitude decried by drug firm boss: investment and new drugs must wait, Pfizer Canada president says. *Vancouver Sun*, January 27: C3.

31 Pharmacare Trends (2001). Pharmacare, Ministry of Health Services. Victoria BC.

32 Graham JR (2001) Reference-based pricing in BC's Pharmacare: a fiscal failure. *Fraser Forum*. May.

33 Bourgault C, Elstein E, Le Lorier J and Suissa S (1999) Reference-based pricing of prescription drugs: exploring the equivalence of angiotensin-converting enzyme inhibitors. *Can Med Assoc J*. **161**: 255–60.

34 Thomas MC, Mann J and Williams S (1998) The impact of reference pricing on clinical lipid control. *NZ Med J*. **111**: 292–4.

35 Zweifel P and Crivelli L (1996) Price regulation of drugs: lessons from Germany. *J Regulatory Economics*. **10**: 257–73.

36 Hazlet TK (1999) *Please, not Another Cadillac: Medicare, pills, and Pharmacare*. Pharmaceutical Outcomes Research & Policy Program. University of Washington, Department of Pharmacy.

37 Lopez-Casasnovas G and Puig-Junoy J (2000) Review of the literature on reference pricing. *Health Policy*. **54**: 87–123.

38 BC Ministry (2000) British Columbia Ministry of Health and Ministry Responsible for Seniors. Briefing note dated April 3.

39 New Zealand Pharmaceuticals Management Agency (PHARMAC) (2001) *Annual Review*. Available from www.pharmac.govt.nz/download/AnnRvw-2001.pdf.

Chapter 16

Disease prevention: the neglected alternative

Norman J. Temple

Why prevention?

Since the 1970s a vast amount of evidence has accumulated demonstrating that the key determinant of the major diseases that afflict Western societies is lifestyle. The essential cause of the great bulk of diseases such as cancer and heart disease lies in the way we choose to conduct our lives – our smoking habits, our diet, and so forth. Based on these discoveries there is now very little debate that most of the diseases that afflict our society are preventable. It is impossible to exaggerate the importance of these medical findings, for they hold the key to effective action for disease prevention at the level of both the individual and the population. This realization inspired the development of many intervention strategies aimed at turning the promise of prevention into a reality.

There are strong reasons in support of a strategy based on prevention. By its very nature, prevention is "low-tech" and should therefore come with a modest price tag. Potentially, far more can be accomplished with far less resources than is typically the case with new "high-tech" treatments. But the advantages of a strategy focused on prevention do not stop there. Even when an effective treatment for a particular disease is available, it is obviously far better if we can prevent that disease, or at least postpone it until later in life. For example, treating a man in his fifties with bypass surgery for severe atherosclerosis will still leave him at high risk of death from heart disease and with reduced quality of life, but primary prevention started years earlier would, in all probability, have given him several extra years of life, free of heart disease.

The clear advantages of a prevention strategy are also demonstrated by taking a historical perspective. Undoubtedly, the most outstanding achievement of biomedical science during the past 150 years was the conquest of many infectious diseases. What is often forgotten is that primary prevention was the driving force behind this great success story. In particular, the widespread adoption of hygiene, after the importance of this was discovered, played a major role. Actual medical treatment, such as the development and use of antibiotics, played a fairly minor role. And if prevention can achieve so much in the war against infectious disease, there is no good reason why a prevention strategy cannot be made to repeat this success story in the war against chronic diseases.

But before looking more closely at the subject of health promotion we shall first take a brief look at some of the evidence that illustrates the enormous potential of a preventive master strategy against chronic diseases.

- Selenium is a mineral present in the diet. Many epidemiological studies have indicated that selenium is protective against various types of cancer.[1,2] More precisely, people whose habitual diet is poor in the mineral are at elevated risk of cancer. One randomized intervention trial has been conducted. This revealed that during the six years of the study, subjects with a poor intake of selenium and who were given a supplement had a much reduced risk of dying of cancer compared with those given placebo.[3,4]
- The Nurses' Health Study is a huge cohort study in which 84 000 American nurses have been tracked for more than 20 years. The investigators carefully examined the risk of coronary heart disease (CHD) in relation to lifestyle. They observed that the 3% of nurses with the healthiest lifestyle have a six times lower risk than the rest of the nurses.[5]
- A study was made of changes in the mortality rate from CHD in Scotland over the years from 1975 to 1994.[6] During this period there were advances in therapy, for example wider use of drug therapy for hypertension, and new developments in drug treatment and surgery for heart disease. At the same time efforts were made to persuade the population to adopt a healthier lifestyle, which is among the least healthy in Europe. Although lifestyle improvements were only modest, this had three times more beneficial impact on CHD (measured as number of life years gained) than did medical and surgical interventions.
- A systematic review of CHD patients revealed that the overall mortality decreases by 36% among those who quit smoking.[7] This decrease is independent of age and gender.
- A study of university alumni examined the relationship between various lifestyle factors and the development of disabilities.[8] The subjects were monitored for 32 years, during which time they went from an average age of 43 to 75. Those with a healthier lifestyle, as indicated by a normal body weight, not smoking, and taking exercise, had a postponement in the development of disabilities of more than five years.

We can also mention here another attractive feature of a healthy lifestyle, namely that it is generally better for the environment. This is because one component of prevention is a reduction in meat consumption. To produce one pound of meat requires about seven pounds of grain as well as a large input of energy, fertilizers, and water. Meat production also requires far more land usage and is suspected of contributing to global warming because the methane produced by cows is a greenhouse gas.

In the remainder of this chapter we explore how the potential of prevention can be translated from the hypothetical to practical reality.

The challenge of prevention

At first glance a prevention strategy could not be simpler: information about the vital importance of good nutrition, exercise, and the avoidance of smoking, is disseminated to members of the public, who are given every encouragement to change their lifestyle, and then, bingo, everyone listens and follows the advice. But, alas, the reality is that despite countless television programs and articles in the print media it has proven extremely difficult to bring about major behavior change at the population level. Certainly, millions have listened to the message and changed their lifestyles to some extent. One area of partial success is smoking. The percentage of Americans who smoked fell from 37.4% in 1970 to 22.5% in 2002.[9] But in most areas the degree of success has been much more modest.

The findings from the following surveys illustrate the wide gap between hope and reality.

- For years Americans have been encouraged to eat "5-a-day" of fruit and vegetables. Between 1972 and 1998, Americans increased their consumption of fruit and vegetables (excluding potatoes) by about one serving per day,[10] an underwhelming rate of progress. Moreover, on any given day half of Americans eat no fruit.[11] In the years 1985–2000 the available food energy in the USA increased by 300 kcal per day. More than 90% of this increased energy came from refined grains, sugars, and added fats, but with a mere 8% coming from fruit and vegetables.[12]
- While millions have taken up exercise, far greater numbers have been left behind. One-third of American adults report no leisure time exercise,[13] while only about one-third achieve an acceptable level of exercise, for example, a brisk walk for at least 30 minutes on most days of the week.[14]
- The British are no better. During the 1990s people in Britain were advised to take regular exercise and eat more healthily. This seems to have had very little impact on the numbers of people taking regular exercise and induced a small increase in consumption of fruit and salads.[15]
- For reasons of both health and appearance no one wants to be overweight. And everyone knows how to take avoiding action: eat less and exercise more. Yet, over the last three decades the USA has been struck by an epidemic of obesity. Between 1976–1980 and 1999–2000 rates of obesity among adults doubled from 14.5% to 30.5%.[16,17] The pandemic of obesity has spread across most Western countries.[18]

Clearly, a preventive approach to medicine holds tremendous potential. But, equally clearly, there are enormous challenges to overcome, especially with respect to a general reluctance of large sections of the population to listen and follow the prevention advice. The rate of progress resembles a severely constipated person who has taken a teaspoon of bran: things are moving, but very slowly.

A number of strategies have been developed over the years in an effort to take the tremendous potential of prevention and use it to improve population health. We shall start by looking at health promotion.

Health promotion campaigns

Starting in the 1970s numerous projects have been carried out in which large numbers of people have been encouraged to lead a healthier lifestyle. The main focus has generally been on the prevention of CHD.

Community-based campaigns

One strategy has been campaigns that have targeted entire communities. Various marketing techniques have been used, such as presentations in schools, displays in supermarkets, and delivering information through the mass media. The degree of success has been mixed.

We will look at three large-scale projects that were carried out in the USA during the 1980s. In each case the aim was to persuade large numbers of people from the target population to exercise more, to cut smoking rates, and to lower elevated levels of blood cholesterol, blood pressure, and weight. The three projects were the Stanford Five-City Project in California,[19] the Pawtucket Heart Health Program in Rhode Island,[20] and the Minnesota Heart Health Program in the Upper Midwest.[21] Over a period of five to eight years diverse methods of behavior modification were used; these included the mass media and education through schools and super-markets. Despite an enormous effort, the results were disappointing. A combined analysis of the results of the three projects revealed that improvements in blood pressure, blood cholesterol, weight, and smoking were of very low magnitude and were not statistically significant.[22] Two more recent community projects also reported a similar lack of success.[23,24]

What went wrong? The most plausible explanation is as follows. These health promotion campaigns took place at a time when large amounts of information were being disseminated, mainly through the mass media, concerning the importance of a healthy lifestyle. As a result millions of Americans were taking steps towards a healthier lifestyle, and rates of CHD were falling. It may be that a health promotion campaign is unlikely to succeed if it takes place against a background of improving lifestyles.

Two European studies may also be mentioned: the German Cardiovascular Prevention Study, conducted from about 1985 to 1992 in the former West Germany,[25] and Action Heart, a community-based health promotion campaign conducted in Rotherham, England, in the early 1990s.[26] In each case a modest degree of success was reported: for example, each study led to a 7% fall in smoking.

Two recent intervention projects represent a radical departure from the strategy used in the above studies. The studies used paid advertising as the major educational tool and aimed to ameliorate just one aspect of lifestyle rather than trying to change several at once. The first study, the 1% Or Less campaign, done in 1996, endeavored to persuade the population of a city in West Virginia to switch from whole milk to low-fat milk.[27] Within just a few weeks sales of low-fat milk, as a proportion of total milk sales, increased from 29% to 46%. This remarkable success was achieved with a budget of under a dollar per person. The second study, carried out in the State of Victoria, Australia from 1992 to 1995, aimed to increase consumption of fruit and vegetables.[28] This was another success story: consumption increased by 11% for fruit and by 17% for vegetables.

Clearly, the results of these attempts to persuade whole communities to improve their lifestyles have been highly variable and often disappointing. More research is required so that consistent success can be achieved in the future. However, we have every reason to suppose that educational approaches at the community level can lead to favorable changes in lifestyle by a fraction of the population and can thereby make at least a modest dent in the burden of chronic disease.

Worksite health promotion

Rather than targeting people at the community level another strategy has been to bring health promotion to the worksite. Quite likely, this appeals to employers as healthier workers are likely to be more productive while sickness-related costs can be expected to decline. Here are some examples of this approach.

The Treatwell program in New England encouraged employees to reduce their fat intake and to increase their intake of dietary fiber.[29] This intervention achieved a small decrease in fat intake (3%) but failed to affect fiber. In the next phase of this program employees and their families were encouraged to increase their intake of fruit and vegetables, and an impressive 19% rise was observed.[30] A project in Minnesota offered weight control and smoking cessation to employees. Compared with control worksites, no change in body weight was detected but the prevalence of smoking was reduced by 2%.[31]

Health promotion as a medical intervention

Another strategy that has been employed is to convey the message in the form of advice in a medical setting. This makes good sense since people are generally receptive to instructions and advice given by doctors and other health professionals. Several such interventions have been carried out.

Two British studies, conducted during the early 1990s, were carried out in the offices of family physicians, with the health advice being given by nurses. In these randomized trials intensive efforts were made to persuade the target groups to follow the lifestyle advice with the goal of reducing risk of cardiovascular disease. The OXCHECK study failed to improve rates of smoking or excessive alcohol intake but did achieve small significant improvements in exercise participation, weight, dietary intake of saturated fat, and blood cholesterol.[32,33] The Family Heart Study reported some modest lifestyle improvements in its target group such that the estimated risk of CHD was reduced by 12%.[34] Overall, therefore, only modest changes were achieved.

Similar findings came from an American study. Patients were given mailed personalized dietary recommendations, educational booklets, a brief physician endorsement, and motivational counseling by telephone. After three months the intervention group had increased its consumption of fruit and vegetables by 0.6 servings per day, but there was no change in intake of red meat or dairy products.[35]

Wilcox and colleagues[36] reviewed 32 intervention studies carried out in a medical setting. They concluded that: "Overall, these interventions tended to produce modest but statistically significant effects for physical activity or exercise, dietary fat, weight loss, blood pressure, and serum cholesterol ... Whereas small by conventional statistical definitions, these findings are likely to be meaningful when considered from a public health perspective."

A variation of the above trials is the targeting of patients at high risk of CHD or other diseases, probably the most cost-effective form of intervention.[37] This strategy has been used with much success in the prevention of type 2 diabetes as demonstrated by the following studies. Two randomized controlled trials were conducted, one in the USA and one in Finland. The subjects were at high risk of the disease because they were overweight and had impaired glucose tolerance.[38,39] The interventions consisted of physical activity and dietary change. In both studies the estimated risk reduction was about 58%, a truly remarkable degree of success. The icing on the cake, so to speak, was that this approach is remarkably cost-effective. The cost per quality-adjusted life year (QALY) in the US study was estimated as a mere $1100 for actual medical expenses, or $8800 when nonmedical costs were included.[40]

In general, interventions focused on high-risk subjects have been more successful than other interventions.[41] Why? First, because the subjects are more likely to follow advice if they realize that the threat to their health is in the not-too-distant future. Second, the same risk factor reduction, for example a modest decrease in blood cholesterol, will prevent more cases of CHD in 100 high-risk subjects than in the same number of low-risk subjects. This is similar to the situation with statins where the cost of preventing a case of CHD falls as the risk of CHD rises. In other words, the prevention of CHD, whether by lifestyle intervention or by using statins, is achieved at lower cost (i.e. dollars per QALY) in those at high risk of CHD than in those at low risk.

But there is more to preventing CHD and other diseases of lifestyle than cost-effectiveness. While the high-risk approach is certainly more cost-effective than giving advice to the entire population, it does have a major deficiency. As Rose[42] pointed out, the 15% of men at "high risk" of CHD account for only 32% of future cases. Therefore, targeting those men only affects a minority of future cases; in order to achieve a major impact on CHD it is necessary to target the entire population. This logic also applies to other diseases related to diet and lifestyle, such as stroke and cancer. In a nutshell, it is the population at a whole that is at risk and in need of lifestyle intervention.

The impact of health promotion

This brief exploration of the world of health promotion reveals that encouraging individuals to change their lifestyles achieves mixed results. Although some projects have been moderately successful, in most cases progress has amounted to no more than a few percentage points. This might be expected to reduce the risk of CHD by about 5% to 15%. While this is certainly beneficial, it will not, however, affect the majority of people at risk. Thus exhortations to the individual, whether via the media, in the community, at the worksite, or in the physician's office, are most unlikely to turn the tide of the Western diseases. Perhaps we can summarize the lesson of health promotion in the words: you can lead a horse to water but you can't make it wear a swimsuit.

But we should not be negative over interventions aimed at encouraging people to improve their lifestyles. On the contrary, minor changes can make valuable contributions to public health that more than justify the expense and effort involved. For instance, Jeffery and associates[31] concluded that a smoking cessation program at a worksite costs about $100 to $200 per smoker who quits (1993 estimate), whereas the cost to the employer for each employee who smokes is far greater. Similarly, Action Heart estimated that the cost per year of life gained was a mere UK£31 (1997 estimate).[26] Health promotion, therefore, can be a cost-effective way to improve lifestyles and thereby improve the health of large numbers of people.[43,44] Indeed, the above comparisons suggest that health promotion can be hundreds of times more cost-effective than such interventions as using statins to prevent heart disease or screening to prevent death from cancer (the cost of those measures was described in previous chapters).

Government policy

Let us now pose the question: Why have health promotion campaigns achieved only modest success? In retrospect, this is not really surprising. There are many factors that shape people's behavior besides concerns about how to stay healthy. Attitudes are affected by factors such as housing, employment, and income. Food purchases are strongly influenced by both price and the advertising to which we are perpetually bombarded. We are also creatures of habit; lifestyle modification is less likely when it requires changes in longstanding behavior and goes against fashion or peer pressure. Another barrier is that individuals have little control over many aspects of their physical environment, such as pollution and food contamination. It is probably naïve, therefore, to expect dramatic results from interventions that merely encourage people to lead a healthier lifestyle.

But this does not mean that we should be resigned to the limited effectiveness of the type of health promotion interventions described above. Rather, we must learn the lessons and formulate a new strategy. Effective interventions will need to tackle the factors that determine why people make choices in the areas relevant to health. What this means in practice is that the central component of new interventions will be policy changes by government.

Governments have the power to pass legislation and to manipulate prices using taxation and subsidies. These government powers have tremendous potential for influencing health behavior.

The effect of price on sales

Action on tobacco control most graphically illustrates the necessity for placing these powers at the service of health promotion. Educational efforts over the last three decades have been enormously important in persuading millions of people to quit smoking. But this still leaves every third or fourth adult in Western countries as a die-hard smoker. There is convincing evidence that price hikes are an effective means to reduce smoking rates. Smoking shows what economists refer to as "price elasticity."[45] It has been estimated that a 10% increase in price reduces tobacco consumption by about 5%, especially among the lower socioeconomic groups.[46] The Canadian experience is particularly illuminating. The prevalence of smoking in young Canadians fell by half during the 1980s in tandem with a doubling of the price. This trend was reversed in the early 1990s when the price was slashed in an attempt to reduce smuggling from the USA.[47]

Studies of the relationship between the price of alcohol and consumption reveal similar price elasticity: a price rise of 10% causes a decrease in consumption of between 3% and 8%.[48]

What applies to tobacco and alcohol also applies to food. Every supermarket manager knows that in order to sell fruit that is becoming overripe quickly, it is necessary to lower the price. From this we can make a critically important inference: the judicious use of taxes and subsidies are a sure means to persuade people to increase their intake of fruit, vegetables, and wholegrain cereals while lowering consumption of less healthy choices, such as foods rich in fat and sugar. This inference is the basis for the blueprint for action proposed here. Recommendations along these lines in the area of food and nutrition policy were advocated by the World Health Organization in 1988.[49]

Evidence confirming the potential of low prices to increase the consumption of healthy food choices comes from a series of studies carried out by Jeffery, French, and colleagues in the USA. In one study the investigators cut by half the price of low-fat snacks sold in vending machines at work sites and secondary schools, and this led to a 93% increase in sales of these foods.[50] In a work site cafeteria the range of fruit and salad ingredients was increased at the same time as the price was halved. As a result purchases trebled.[51] A similar study conducted in a high school cafeteria produced much the same result.[52]

Advertising, marketing, and labeling of food

Food advertising probably exerts a major influence on people's diets.[53] After all, the fact that commercial enterprises, large and small, spend so lavishly on advertising is eloquent testimony to its effectiveness. It is scarcely surprising, therefore, that health promotion campaigns achieve such poor levels of success when they must compete against ubiquitous advertising of unhealthy food choices. For example, the annual advertising budgets in the USA in 2003 for Coca-Cola, Burger King, and McDonald's were $473 million, $524 million, and $619 million, respectively.[54] This dwarfs the million dollars a year spent by the National Cancer Institute on the education component of its 5-a-day campaign to promote fruit and vegetable consumption. Overall, only about 2.2% of the food advertising budget is used to promote consumption of healthy foods such as fruits, vegetables, whole grains, and beans.[55]

Food advertisers spare no effort to win the hearts and mouths of children to junk food. An American study of advertisements appearing on Saturday morning TV found that the vast majority were for such foods as highly-sugared cereals, fast-food restaurants, and the like, while none were for fruit and vegetables.[56] A study published in 2005 showed that very little has changed during the previous decade: 83% of foods ads promoted foods of low nutritional value.[57] The situation in Canada is little different.[58]

Advertising is but one part of the wider production and marketing strategy of the food industry. For example, in response to the demand for low-fat foods, manufacturers sell foods with less fat, but the missing fat often reappears in foods that are often little more than concoctions of fat, sugar, and salt.[59] The problem is compounded by the fact that food labeling is confusing to most consumers.

Government policy and food

The above discussion points to the conclusion that government policies, concerning food prices and, to a lesser extent, food advertising and labeling, may be an effective means to help bring about desirable changes in eating patterns. Here are some specific proposals as to how government policies could be modified along these lines.[60,61]

- Subsidies paid to milk producers could be changed to favor low-fat milk. Likewise, by the use of tools such as subsidies, taxation, and labeling, the sale of fruit juice could be encouraged over sugar-rich soft drinks and of low-fat meat over high-fat varieties.

- There is much scope for improved food labels so as to help consumers more easily purchase foods with a low content of fat, especially saturated fat. In addition, labeling and nutrition information should be extended to areas presently exempt from food labels, especially restaurant menus and fresh meat.
- Schools should be compelled to restrict the sale of junk food. Where meals are provided, these should be of superior health value. Similar policies could be applied to other institutions under government control, such as the military, prisons, and cafeterias in government offices.
- Television advertising could be regulated so as to control the content, duration, and frequency of commercials for unhealthy food products, especially when the target audience is children.

This strategy can be applied to other areas of lifestyle. As discussed above, it is well established that a hike in prices is especially effective at tackling the curse of smoking. In particular, it protects young people from their immaturity. Another area requiring government intervention is advertising: unlike many other countries the USA still allows advertising for cigarettes in magazines. Similarly, policy initiatives can be used to encourage more people to exercise. Many people are discouraged from taking exercise because of the various barriers that exist, such as lack of appropriate facilities, high membership fees at gyms, and roads that are too dangerous for bikes. Here government policies could directly tackle these barriers.

There seems to have been considerably more discussion of these general ideas in recent years. One factor, more so than any other, appears to be sparking a change in the area of nutrition policy, namely the ever-expanding pandemic of obesity. Given the dismal record of both health education and of therapeutic medicine in their dealings with this condition, it is probably inevitable that radical ideas will now be seriously discussed.

The public health policies proposed above are best seen as nothing more than a logical extension of those already well established. The use of seat belts is a good example of how a law can save lives at little cost and with minimal intrusion into individual freedom. Lead pollution is another excellent illustration of what can be achieved by governmental action. In the 1970s regulations implemented by the American government forced major reductions or removal of lead from gasoline, paint, water, and consumer products. As a result there was a four-fold reduction in the average blood lead level of American children over the following 20 years.[62,63]

Barriers against public health policies

One obvious objection that might be made against public health policies is that they somehow infringe on personal liberties. But this seems like a weak argument. The issues of seat belt use and drink driving illustrate that when legislation is implemented and the public is educated as to its importance, there is a high degree of acceptance. Likewise, across the Western world the public has seldom voiced much protest against "sin" taxes on alcohol and cigarettes.

A major obstacle to the implementation of public health policies is that industries that profit from unhealthy lifestyles use their considerable resources to resist change. Time and time again we find examples of industries lobbying governments and throwing their money around in order to delay, dilute, or stop laws that threaten their profits. And, more often than not, governments show more sympathy for the financial demands of industry than for the health needs of the general public. Indeed, the unrestrained free market ideology that has gained enormous influence over the past quarter-century means that governments have become ever more business friendly and noninterventionist than ever.

The tobacco industry provides the starkest illustration of this. The US Congress has been very lethargic when it comes to antismoking legislation. Researchers investigated the likely reason for this and concluded that: "The money that the tobacco industry donates to members of Congress ensures that the tobacco industry will retain its strong influence in the federal tobacco policy process."[64]

What is true for the tobacco industry is equally true for the agricultural and food industries. Typically, while the health arm of governments encourages people to eat less fat, the departments responsible for the agricultural and food industries are largely concerned with maintaining high sales. Philip James and Ann Ralph[59] from Scotland asserted that: "Analysis of different policies suggests that health issues are readily squeezed out of discussion by economic and vested interests." There is considerable evidence of how industry has successfully pressured governments to bow to their wishes on questions of nutrition policy. The history of this in the USA is detailed in a book by Marion Nestle[65] of New York University, *Food Politics. How the Food Industry Influences Nutrition and Health*.

Almost everyone consumes a greatly excessive amount of salt, most of which is added by manufacturers to processed food.[66] This salt plays a role in several diseases, especially hypertension and stroke. However, food manufacturers have opposed attempts to reduce the salt content of food. Discussing this question Fiona Goodlee,[67] assistant editor of the *BMJ*, put it as follows:

> ... *some of the world's major food manufacturers have adopted desperate measures to try to stop governments from recommending salt reduction. Rather than reformulate their products, manufacturers have lobbied governments, refused to cooperate with expert working parties, encouraged misinformation campaigns, and tried to discredit the evidence ... The tactics over salt are much the same as those used by other sectors of industry. The Sugar Association in the United States and the Sugar Bureau in Britain have waged fierce campaigns against links between sugar and obesity and dental caries.*

The cost-effectiveness of health promotion

This chapter has explored various forms of health promotion. Here we examine whether this is a cost-effective approach to improving population heath, especially when we bear in mind the meager success rate of many interventions.

First, we need to explore some basic principles of the cost-effectiveness of prevention. It would be a mistake to see the prevention of fatal cases of heart disease and cancer as "saving" lives. Rather, each such case is, in reality, a death postponed. A dollar saved today in preventing a case of heart disease or cancer will likely mean a dollar (perhaps more) spent at a later time for treatment of a chronic nonfatal disease followed by death from cancer or stroke. In other words, prevention typically postpones rather than reduces healthcare expenditures. The great advantage of prevention lies not in reduced healthcare costs but elsewhere: it adds years to life and life to years. And that, of course, is precisely what medicine is supposed to be all about.

Let us start with public health policies. You do not need to have taken Health Economics 101 to figure out that policy approaches to health promotion will, in most cases, cost little or nothing. For example, governments could easily force food manufacturers to slash the salt content of food. Few actions would achieve so much at virtually no cost. If taxes and subsidies were realigned so that health became the top priority, this could be revenue neutral. Extra costs in some areas (such as subsidies for fruit and whole grain cereals; making cities more bike friendly) would be cancelled out by increased income in other areas (for example, higher taxes on cigarettes and sugar-rich soft drinks).

But what about other forms of health promotion, those based on providing education and encouragement? In order to make meaningful comparisons with medical interventions, we must make comparisons in terms of the cost of generating QALYs, as described in Chapter 1. On this basis, health promotion is, generally speaking, a cost-effective means to generate QALYs.

When physicians give advice to their patients to quit smoking, the response rate is very low, a mere 2% or so. Nevertheless, this is still a highly cost-effective intervention: the estimated cost of preventing one death by this means is a mere $1500 (1995 estimate).[68] As quitting smoking will, on average, add several years to the life of a smoker, the cost per QALY is a mere few hundred dollars. A 1997 estimate put the cost of smoking cessation interventions at $1555 per QALY.[69] Other researchers estimated the cost of a school-based antismoking intervention.[70] Although the numbers are very imprecise, the best guess is $20 000 per QALY. It seems reasonable to assume that as different types of interventions are developed and tested, the effectiveness of educational interventions will improve, and the cost per QALY will decrease.

Studies have been made of the cost-effectiveness of various forms of health promotion. A major review concluded that each dollar spent on health promotion results in savings of two or three dollars in reduced absenteeism and about three to six dollars in reduced healthcare costs.[43] Most of the studies looked at in this review were carried out at the worksite over just a few years. The benefits were therefore attributed to short-term effects, such as less stress, rather than the prevention of diseases that take decades to develop, such as CHD and cancer.

While more study is clearly required as to the cost-effectiveness of various forms of health promotion, we can be optimistic that this strategy compares very favorably with more conventional medical interventions.

Conclusion

Health promotion is clearly a work in progress. It has enormous potential but considerably more research is required.[71] We may be confident that future research will reveal how more effective interventions may be carried out. Nevertheless, we are already at the stage where health promotion is a cost-effective tool for improving the health of millions of people. The time is long overdue for prevention to lose its Cinderella status and be invited to the ball.

What is very clear is that interventions based on encouraging people to change their lifestyle, while commendable and worthwhile, are likely to be far less effective than actions carried out by governments in the form of manipulating taxes and subsidies, and by the use of various policy initiatives. There is clearly a serious need for a change in the mindset of the key players.

References

1   Zhuo H, Smith AH and Steinmaus C (2004) Selenium and lung cancer: a quantitative analysis of heterogeneity in the current epidemiological literature. *Cancer Epidemiol Biomarkers Prev.* 13: 771–8.

2   Li H, Stampfer MJ, Giovannucci EL *et al.* (2004) A prospective study of plasma selenium levels and prostate cancer risk. *J Natl Cancer Inst.* 96: 696–703.

3   Clark LC, Combs GF, Turnbull BW *et al.* (1996) Effects of selenium supplementation for cancer prevention in patients with carcinoma of the skin. A randomized trial. *JAMA.* 276: 1957–63.

4   Duffield-Lillico AJ, Reid ME, Turnbull BW *et al.* (2002) Baseline characteristics and the effect of selenium supplementation on cancer incidence in a randomized clinical trial: a summary report of the Nutritional Prevention of Cancer Trial. *Cancer Epidemiol Biomarkers Prev.* 11: 630–9.

5   Stampfer MJ, Hu FB, Manson JE, Rimm EB and Willett WC (2000) Primary prevention of coronary heart disease in women through diet and lifestyle. *N Engl J Med.* 343: 16–22.

6   Critchley JA, Capewell S and Unal B (2003) Life-years gained from coronary heart disease mortality reduction in Scotland: prevention or treatment? *J Clin Epidemiol.* 56: 583–90.

7   Critchley JA and Capewell S (2003) Mortality risk reduction associated with smoking cessation in patients with coronary heart disease: a systematic review. *JAMA.* 290: 86–97.

8   Vita AJ, Terry RB, Hubert HB and Fries JF (1998) Aging, health risks, and cumulative disability. *N Engl J Med.* 338: 1035–41.

9   National Center for Chronic Disease Prevention and Health Promotion. Smoking Prevalence Among U.S. Adults. Available from www.cdc.gov/tobacco/research_data/adults_prev/prevali (accessed January 11, 2005).

10 Krebs-Smith SM and Kantor LS (2001) Choose a variety of fruits and vegetables daily: understanding the complexities. *J Nutr.* 131 (2S-1): 487S–501S.

11 Tippett KS and Cleveland LE (1999) Cited in: Frazao E, America's eating habits: changes and consequences. USDA/ERS, *Agricultural Information Bulletin.* 750: 51–70.

12 Putnam J, Allshouse J and Kantor LS (2002) U.S. per capita food supply trends: more calories, refined carbohydrates, and fats. *Food Review.* 25: 2–15.

13 Anon (1998) Self-reported physical inactivity by degree of urbanization – United States, 1996. *MMWR Morb Mortal Wkly Rep.* 47: 1097–100.

14 Jones DA, Ainsworth BE, Croft JB, Macera CA, Lloyd EE and Yusuf HR (1998) Moderate leisure-time physical activity: who is meeting the public health recommendations? A national cross-sectional study. *Arch Fam Med.* 7: 285–9.

15 Parsons TJ, Manor O and Power C (2005) Changes in diet and physical activity in the 1990s in a large British sample (1958 birth cohort). *Eur J Clin Nutr.* 59: 49–56.

16 Flegal KM, Carroll MD, Kuczmarski RJ and Johnson CL (1998) Overweight and obesity in the United States: prevalence and trends, 1960–1994. *Int J Obesity.* 22: 39–47.

17 Flegal KM, Carroll MD, Ogden CL and Johnson CL (2002) Prevalence and trends in obesity among US adults, 1999–2000. *JAMA.* 288: 1723–7.

18 Siedell JC (1995) Obesity in Europe: scaling an epidemic. *Int J Obesity.* 19 (Suppl. 3): S1–S4.

19 Farquhar JW, Fortmann SP, Flora JA *et al.* (1990) Effects of communitywide education on cardiovascular disease risk factors. The Stanford Five-City Project. *JAMA.* 264: 359–65.

20 Carleton RA, Lasater TM, Assaf AR *et al.* (1995) The Pawtucket Heart Health Program: community changes in cardiovascular risk factors and projected disease risk. *Am J Public Health.* 85: 777–85.

21 Luepker RV, Murray DM, Jacobs DR *et al.* (1994) Community education for cardiovascular disease prevention: risk factor changes in the Minnesota Heart Health Program. *Am J Public Health.* 84: 1383–93.

22 Winkleby MA, Feldman HA and Murray DM (1994) Joint analysis of three U.S. community intervention trials for reduction of cardiovascular risk. *J Clin Epidemiol.* **50**: 645–58.

23 Goodman RM, Wheeler FC and Lee PR (1995) Evaluation of the Heart To Heart Project: lessons from a community-based chronic disease prevention project. *Am J Health Promot.* **9**: 443–55.

24 Brownson RC, Smith CA, Pratt M *et al.* (1996) Preventing cardiovascular disease through community-based risk reduction: the Bootheel Heart Health Project. *Am J Public Health.* **86**: 206–13.

25 Hoffmeister H, Mensink GB, Stolzenberg H *et al.* (1996) Reduction of coronary heart disease risk factors in the German Cardiovascular Prevention study. *Prev Med.* **25**: 135–45.

26 Baxter T, Milner P, Wilson K *et al.* (1997) A cost effective, community based heart health promotion project in England: prospective comparative study. *BMJ.* **315**: 582–5.

27 Reger B, Wootan MG and Booth-Butterfield S (1999) Using mass media to promote healthy eating: a community-based demonstration project. *Prev Med.* **29**: 414–21.

28 Dixon H, Boland R, Segan C, Stafford H and Sindall C (1998) Public reaction to Victoria's "2 Fruit 'n' 5 Veg Day" campaign and reported consumption of fruit and vegetables. *Prev Med.* **27**: 572–82.

29 Sorensen G, Morris DM, Hunt MK *et al.* (1992) Work-site nutrition intervention and employees' dietary habits: the Treatwell program. *Am J Public Health.* **82**: 877–80.

30 Sorensen G, Stoddard A, Peterson K *et al.* (1999) Increasing fruit and vegetable consumption through worksites and families in the Treatwell 5-a-Day Study. *Am J Public Health.* **89**: 54–60.

31 Jeffery RW, Forster JL, French SA *et al.* (1993) The Healthy Worker Project: a work-site intervention for weight control and smoking cessation. *Am J Public Health.* **83**: 395–401.

32 Imperial Cancer Research Fund OXCHECK Study Group (1994) Effectiveness of health checks conducted by nurses in primary care: results of the OXCHECK study after one year. *BMJ.* **308**: 308–12.

33 Imperial Cancer Research Fund OXCHECK Study Group (1995) Effectiveness of health checks conducted by nurses in primary care: final results of the OXCHECK study. *BMJ.* **310**: 1099–104.

34 Family Heart Study Group (1994) Randomised controlled trial evaluating cardiovascular screening and intervention in general practice: principal results of British Family Heart Study. *BMJ.* **308**: 313–20.

35 Delichatsios HK, Hunt MK, Lobb R, Emmons K and Gillman MW (2001) EatSmart: efficacy of a multifaceted preventive nutrition intervention in clinical practice. *Prev Med.* 33 (2 Pt 1): 91–8.

36 Wilcox S, Parra-Medina D, Thompson-Robinson M and Will J (2001) Nutrition and physical activity interventions to reduce cardiovascular disease risk in health care settings: a quantitative review with a focus on women. *Nutr Rev.* **59**: 197–214.

37 Field K, Thorogood M, Silagy C, Normand C, O'Neill C and Muir J (1995) Strategies for reducing coronary risk factors in primary care: which is most cost effective? *BMJ.* **310**: 1109–12.

38 Tuomilehto J, Lindstrom J, Eriksson JG *et al.* (2001) Prevention of type 2 diabetes mellitus by changes in lifestyle among subjects with impaired glucose tolerance. *N Engl J Med.* **344**: 1343–50.

39 Knowler WC, Barrett-Connor E, Fowler SE *et al.* (2002) Reduction in the incidence of type 2 diabetes with lifestyle intervention or metformin. *N Engl J Med.* **346**: 393–403.

40 Herman WH, Hoerger TJ, Brandle M *et al.* (2005) The cost-effectiveness of lifestyle modification or metformin in preventing type 2 diabetes in adults with impaired glucose tolerance. *Ann Intern Med.* **142**: 323–32.

41 Ammerman AS, Lindquist CH, Lohr KN and Hersey J (2002) The efficacy of behavioral interventions to modify dietary fat and fruit and vegetable intake: a review of the evidence. *Prev Med.* **35**: 25–41.

42 Rose G (1992) *The Strategy of Preventive Medicine.* Oxford University Press, Oxford.

43 Aldana SG (2001) Financial impact of health promotion programs: a comprehensive review of the literature. *Am J Health Promot.* **15**: 296–320.

44 Golaszewski T (2001) Shining lights: studies that have most influenced the understanding of health promotion's financial impact. *Am J Health Promot.* **15**: 332–40.

45 Meier KJ and Licari MJ (1997) The effect of cigarette taxes on cigarette consumption, 1955 through 1994. *Am J Public Health.* **87**: 1126–30.

46   Townsend J (1996) Price and consumption of tobacco. *Br Med Bull.* **52**: 132–42.
47   Stephens T, Pedersen LL, Koval JJ and Kim C (1997) The relationship of cigarette prices and no-smoking bylaws to the prevalence of smoking in Canada. *Am J Public Health.* **87**: 1519–21.
48   Anderson P and Lehto G (1994) Prevention policies. *Br Med Bull.* **50**: 171–85.
49   World Health Organization Regional Office for Europe (1988) *The Adelaide Recommendations: healthy public policy regional office for Europe.* World Health Organization, Geneva.
50   French SA, Jeffery RW, Story M *et al.* (2001) Pricing and promotion effects on low-fat vending snack purchases: the CHIPS Study. *Am J Public Health.* **91**: 112–17.
51   Jeffery RW, French SA, Raether C and Baxter JE (1994) An environmental intervention to increase fruit and salad purchases in a cafeteria. *Prev Med.* **23**: 788–92.
52   French SA, Story M, Jeffery RW *et al.* (1997) Pricing strategy to promote fruit and vegetable purchase in high school cafeterias. *J Am Diet Assoc.* **97**: 1008–10.
53   Nestle M, Wing R, Birch L *et al.* (1998) Behavioral and social influence on food choice. *Nutr Rev.* **56**: S50–S64.
54   Advertising Age (2004) *Advertising Age. 100 Leading National Advertisers: 49th Annual Report.* June 28.
55   Gallo AE (1999) Food advertising in the United States. In: Frazao E, ed. *America's Eating Habits: changes and consequences.* USDA, Washington, DC.
56   Kotz K and Story M (1994) Food advertisements during children's Saturday morning television programming: Are they consistent with dietary recommendations? *J Am Diet Assoc.* **94**: 1296–300.
57   Harrison K and Marske AL (2005) Nutritional content of foods advertised during the television programs children watch most. *Am J Public Health.* **95**: 1568–74.
58   Ostbye T, Pomerleau, White M, Coolich M and McWhinney J (1993) Food and nutrition in Canadian "prime time" television commercials. *Can J Public Health.* **84**: 370–4.
59   James WPT and Ralph A (1992) National strategies for dietary change. In: Marmot M and Elliott P, eds. *Coronary Heart Disease. From Aetiology to Public Health.* Oxford University Press, Oxford.
60   Nestle M and Jacobson MF (2000) Halting the obesity epidemic: a public health policy approach. *Public Health Rep.* **115**: 12–24.
61   Jacobson MF and Brownell KD (2000) Small taxes on soft drinks and snack foods to promote health. *Am J Public Health.* **90**: 854–7.
62   Pirkle JL, Brody DJ, Gunter EW *et al.* (1994) The decline in blood lead levels in the United States. *JAMA.* **272**: 284–91.
63   Brody DJ, Pirkle JL, Kramer RA *et al.* (1994) Blood lead levels in the U.S. population. *JAMA.* **272**: 277–83.
64   Moore S, Wolfe SM, Lindes D and Douglas CE (1994) Epidemiology of failed tobacco control legislation. *JAMA.* **272**: 1171–5.
65   Nestle M (2002) *Food Politics. How the Food Industry Influences Nutrition and Health.* University of California Press, Berkeley, CA.
66   Kaplan NM (2000) Evidence in favor of moderate dietary sodium reduction. *Am J Hypertens.* **13**: 8–13.
67   Goodlee F (1996) The food industry fights for salt. *BMJ.* **312**: 1239–40.
68   Law M and Tang JL (1995) An analysis of the effectiveness of interventions intended to help people stop smoking. *Arch Intern Med.* **155**: 1933–41.
69   Cromwell J, Bartosch WJ and Mitchell JB (1997) *The Cost-effectiveness of AHCPR's Smoking Cessation Guideline.* US Department of Health and Human Services, Public Health Service, Agency for Health Care Policy and Research, Rockville, MD; AHCPR publication 97-R049.
70   Tengs TO, Osgood ND and Chen LL (2001) The cost-effectiveness of intensive national school-based anti-tobacco education: results from the tobacco policy model. *Prev Med.* **33**: 558–70.
71   Finkelstein E, French S, Variyam JN and Haines PS (2004) Pros and cons of proposed interventions to promote healthy eating. *Am J Prev Med.* **27** (Suppl.): 163–71.

Chapter 17

Promoting the health of the medical profession: environmentalism and commercialism in medical education

Iahn Gonsenhauser, Danny George, and Peter J. Whitehouse

Introduction

Throughout its history the medical profession has struggled to find a balance between maintaining the status quo and adapting to meet the needs of society. Talk of professional control and commitment to reform has often been overpowered by externally imposed forces of change. Medical schools often talk of reform but do very little changing.[1] According to Kenneth Ludmerer[2] one medical school dean stated: "There's an enormous gap between talking about educational changes and accomplishing them." Ludmerer also pointed to the sociologist Samuel Bloom as having referred to this as "reform without change."

It has been 100 years since the most influential reorganization of medical education in North America. At that time, medicine shifted from business-practical to more academic-analytical methods of instruction, represented by the creation of the Council on Medical Education at the American Medical Association and the improvement of American medical education known as the "Flexnerian Revolution."[3] Abraham Flexner is credited with inciting the revolutionary revamping of medical education in the USA as a result of his 1910 report for the Carnegie Foundation for the Advancement of Teaching, *Medical Education in the United States and Canada*, which exposed the rampant commercialism and poor standards of education in medical schools at the time.[3] The motivating force for Flexner was one of concern for public health. He is quoted as having said that the exploitation of medicine at the time was "strangely inconsistent with the social aspects of medical practice. The overwhelming importance of preventive medicine, sanitation, and public health indicates that in modern life the medical profession is an organ differentiated by society for its highest purpose, not a business to be exploited."[4]

We find ourselves again facing revolutionary change in medicine. Over the past few decades, the influence of managed-care organizations on medicine has begun to radically change its structure and practice, as well as medical education.[5] As a result medical schools have become more dependent on a recent outpouring of research dollars from the National Institute of Health (NIH) and industry. The financial support for medical education, often subsidized by the "profits" of research and clinical care, has been further weakened. During the same time, the size of medical school faculties has increased and the investment in facilities has also increased. Physicians find themselves needing to see more patients to sustain their practices, leaving less time for teaching, as well as less time to see individual patients. "The clinical education of medical students is often dependent on busy residents and fellows still in training themselves or part-time clinical faculty."[2]

Financial pressures are now affecting medical education in dramatic ways. The reorganization of healthcare in the USA is still in turmoil, and is driven by rising costs. Managed care, clinical guidelines, the large number of uninsured patients, and pharmacoeconomic issues are slowly forcing major changes in the business of medicine. As Ludmerer[2] said:

> By the late 1990s, a second revolutionary period in American medical education had begun. Under pressure from HMOs, academic health centers were increasingly unable to use clinical revenues to cross-subsidize education, research, and charity care, and managed care's mandate to treat patients quickly was wreaking havoc on a learning environment whose essential characteristic was time. More subtle but equally pernicious, academic health centers were losing the market for their educational products, as the new managed-care environment was making it increasingly difficult for doctors to practice in concordance with many traditional professional teachings and values.

The current form of medical education is no longer sustainable, and issues of public health and prevention have once again been thrust to the forefront of medicine. The challenge we face today is in providing answers to both the financial obstacles present in educating our future physicians, and adjusting our focus to more directly attend to issues of professionalism and standards of care that include global and community health.

Medical education today is too narrowly focused on individual health and reductionist molecular science. The genetic revolution, which was discussed in Chapter 10, promises new drugs tailored to individual diseases, defined by increasingly precise nosologies, to individual patients through pharmacogenomics. This promise of so-called personalized medicine may, however, be both depersonalizing and false. Do patients want to be defined by their genes, rather than their stories? Do they want their medical histories to better reflect the values in their own lives? Do the promises that commercialized medicine makes offer too much false hope?

The definition of medical professionalism is being revised to address these concerns. The social contract that was once limited in scope to the care of individual patients is now being reevaluated and passed on through new pedagogies to enlighten medical students to the social, ethical, economic, and environmental issues facing human health. Medical professionalism, seen in this new light, requires a more holistic understanding of medical practice as a part of a broader social context. This broader social fabric weaves together issues such as the increasing harm caused by toxic chemicals from the environment, infectious agents, and climate change, the politics of healthcare, and the biases imposed by industry interests on medical research and practice. Although we are suggesting more public health-inclusive ideals, they cannot be successful if they are achieved at the expense of the focus on individual patient care. The future of societal health lies in balancing these important approaches.

In the remainder of this chapter we illustrate our concerns by highlighting the neglected topic of nutrition in medical school curricula. We describe briefly how our medical school, Case Western Reserve University, in Cleveland, Ohio, is trying to address broader issues concerning health in its current efforts at curriculum change. We use obesity and nutritional knowledge as an example of how clinical and population medicine must work together to promote both individual and community health. We end by describing a proposed medical school elective to broaden students' (and faculty's) conceptions of environmental health and how commercial influences affect personal and community health.

The escalating prevalence of obesity in adults and children has been called an epidemic.[6] The metabolic syndrome incorporates dyslipidemia, elevated blood pressure, impaired glucose tolerance, and obesity. This group of symptoms is poised to overtake cigarette smoking as the leading cause of heart disease in the USA.[7] The primary treatment in battling the metabolic syndrome is weight loss, but people can benefit simply from increased physical activity or decreased caloric intake even in the absence of weight loss. Some benefit in cases of metabolic syndrome would also be generated by increasing fruit and vegetable intake, along with increasing the consumption of whole grains and low-fat dairy foods; however, certain aspects of the culture in the USA, notably portion size,[8,9] food preference,[6,10,11] and the sedentary nature of both work and leisure[7,11,12] undermine these treatment options and represent a general hindrance to the practice of prevention and nutrition. When physicians make attempts at incorporating these concepts into practice, patient compliance is often difficult to achieve, and the fact that physicians have less and less time to devote to individual patients for encouraging lifestyle changes makes it more difficult still.

An additional problem is that most physicians are not armed with the knowledge necessary to effectively implement these practices, and are therefore unaware of how to affect their patients. We need to teach not only how to think as medical professionals, but how to act. To learn about prevention in relation to diet and exercise, for example, means more than just adding courses on nutrition and exercise physiology. In order to be effective, medical students must learn how to influence the behavior of both patients and communities, in addition to technical knowledge, so that they can later, as physicians, provide practical strategies.

The University of Pennsylvania, School of Medicine, has implemented a program promoting the inclusion of nutrition and prevention in medical education. Its mission – "To engage medical students and residents in active learning about nutrition through a multidisciplinary, integrated, medical education curriculum" – has led to the total integration of nutrition curriculum goals into the general medical education, known as Curriculum 2000.[13] The UPENN model addresses the need for nutrition as a focus, but fails to address the broader, more challenging issue of redefining medical professionalism. Other medical schools are implementing curriculum changes that incorporate nutrition and prevention, as well as attending to the need to revise the societal role and responsibilities of medicine. Case Western Reserve University is currently revising its curriculum and considering renaming its School of Medicine as the School of Medicine *and Health*.[1]

At Case a new focus on research pertaining to proteomics, metabolomics, and genomics as well as public health is emerging through the development of an Institute for Patient and Population Sciences. This institute will foster technology transfer involving both basic biological and epidemiological sciences. Phrases like "tearing down silos" and "spiraling" refer to attempts now being made to place greater emphasis on cross-disciplinary topics. Medical school curriculum planners are attempting to incorporate nutrition by integrating basic science principles into general coursework in biochemistry and gastrointestinal medicine, and transform these basic science principles into relevant and applicable practices. Schools of medicine are hoping to enable physicians to process information in more insightful and critical ways.

Although it is clear that basic nutrition has been an underutilized topic in physicians' training, and efforts are being made to change this, there are still issues beyond the curriculum that hamper this effort. There is little, if any, knowledge of nutrition required to successfully navigate medical board examinations. This is a key factor in motivating any medical school to incorporate these concepts into its curriculum. Academic incentives to encourage faculty to focus on teaching, in particular teaching these topics, are needed. A vast discontinuity exists between basic science researchers in the fields of biochemistry or nutrition and clinical practitioners, whose responsibility it is to implement these concepts into practice. In examples of successful medical education, clinical training parallels theoretical or conceptual teaching. In order to offer a consistent training this technology/informational transfer chasm must be bridged.

Part of the future scope of medicine is enabling physicians to incorporate new learning about prevention, nutrition, and public health into their practices. Another aspect of this is teaching them about the importance of environmental factors in health, and the role of those industries whose environmental impacts affect us (and not only the pharmaceutical and health industries). Medicine today seems dominated by one easily measured value – money. It is time to revive other values in the medical profession. An important one is respect for nature. The social contract between medicine and society is being renegotiated. In the course description that follows we seek to improve physicians' understanding of how money has distorted healthcare and how allying with nature can enhance human and ecological health.

In order to respond to this need for education about environmental and commercial concerns, we have designed a new medical school elective entitled ''The World of the Healer,'' which we now describe.

The world of the healer

Dean Ralph Horowitz of Case Western Reserve University has issued the statement that the focus of the School of Medicine will be to prepare physicians who are devoted to the biology of disease and the social determinants of illness, the care of individual patients, and the health of the public.[1] This statement very broadly encompasses what many physicians and educators believe are the true values of medical professionalism. It is also an appropriate response to the recent criticism directed at medical schools for their failure to instill in students knowledge of a more contemporary ''social contract'' linking healers and communities. The statement also reflects the need to respond to the cynicism and pessimism that develops during medical education, which, in turn, erodes the social and human value so necessary for effective medical practice.

Course outline

In the ''World of the Healer'' course we implement an elective that guides medical students through content, dialogue, and reflection which, through their own narrative journey, helps them arrive at an understanding of what medical professionalism truly is. To do so, we seek to create an environment of open communication, free of recrimination and reproach. This environment is intended to offer a reprieve from the typically judgmental and competitive surroundings that deter most students from offering compassion and support to their peers in medical school. We hope that by establishing this opportunity for open and candid dialogue, the students will engage in the creation and sharing of collective wisdom about what the core values of medical professionalism are.

The overall course objectives are as follows.

- To elucidate the meaning of "professionalism" in medicine, in the context of environmental health and medical commerce.
- To understand, through the exchange of personal stories, the role of money in medicine and to discuss how money and "profit motive" may affect professional values.
- To explore how business can both damage and improve the environment, thereby affecting health, either negatively or positively.
- To discover how we relate to our natural environmental systems, and to affirm our responsibility for community health, as well as the health of our individual patients.
- To reaffirm our commitment as society's healers, and to rediscover the heart and soul of medical service in the context of our healthcare organizations.

This course is a collection of five two-hour sessions, each of value as a stand-alone seminar on a particular issue, but together offering a transformative experience. There is no testing or grading, but students will be asked to complete a self-assessment and course evaluation. Pass/fail grading is intended, with passing marks contingent on attendance and participation.

Selections from a course reader, comprising a collection of academic and literary readings, are recommended but not required for each session. The session discussions focus on individual experiences. In keeping with the principle of open, equal, and comfortable sharing, each of the five World of the Healer sessions begins with an informal "conversation starter" presented by a facilitator. This is intended to allow students to begin to develop their own thoughts on the session's focus so that they will be able to participate in the discussions.

Topics covered include: the direct impact of commercialism on medicine; the impact of commercialism on nature and the implications that this impact poses on health and healthcare; what medicine's obligation to the environment is; and how organizations can be better prepared and motivated to address their social responsibilities. The path of this curriculum is intended to spiral outward from our first session in that we will begin by defining professions and medical professionalism and terminate with the creation of mission statements for medical professional organizations which include these definitions and address the obstacles that face them.

Ideology and the medical profession

In our first session we begin by broadly defining profession and professionalism. The definition Reynolds[14] reaches is as follows: "Medical professionalism is a set of values, attitudes, and behaviors that results in serving the interests of patients and society before one's own." For our purposes this definition fits well but is not adequate in addressing the "ism" of professionalism. For students of medicine, understanding the abstract definition of medical professionalism is not enough. Without an understanding of how the concept is shaped and defined, and what their responsibility as stewards of medical professionalism is, they remain external from a concept which they seemingly aspire to be a part of. "Isms" take specific concepts and refer to all actions or processes regarding them.[15] A medical professional acts in accordance to the code of conduct created by the medical community. One who practices medical professionalism is engaged in virtuous professional actions that serve to support and define the meaning of the title "medical professional."

Our intention is that by the end of the first session, students will identify not just the code of conduct and values associated with being a medical professional (altruism, accountability, excellence, duty to service, integrity, respect, empathy, compassion, and lifelong education) but also the responsibility on their part to continually assess and adjust this set of values and behaviors through their own actions.

We will focus on defining profession and briefly summarize what values underlie the medical profession. Students will produce their own sets of values for medicine and discuss how these values are formed. We will define professionalism and discuss what values anchor professionalism in medicine.

Commercialism and medicine

During session two, the effect of commercialism, or profit-driven medicine, will be explored. Specifically, we will focus on the influence of academic–industry relationships (AIRs) on medical practice and research. It is in AIRs that we find some of the toughest obstacles facing nutrition and prevention. It would be easy to pay attention only to conflict of interest and deficiencies in ethics, but we will also give credence to the benefits reaped by medicine through its relationship with industry.

The consanguinity of medicine and industry is an important point. Were it not for the pecuniary aspects of the business of medicine, the height to which the industry has grown may never have been achieved. As evidenced by the practice of many physicians, health promotion has not been the primary function of medicine. It is for the sake of distinguishing the ideal nature and purpose of medicine versus the nature of private industry that we separate the two; however, it is imperative to acknowledge the reciprocating nature of the disciplines.

In session two we examine the question of how money influences medicine and the dilemma that is AIR. On the one hand, industry is responsible for a great deal of financial backing in the sciences. In fact, the American Association for the Advancement of Science states that while federal support for "health-related" research has increased from $2 billion in the 1960s to slightly less than $16 billion in 1998, private-sector research has grown from approximately $2 billion to an estimated $21.1 billion during that period.[16] The amount of funding received through private industry clearly reflects the necessity for science to maintain this relationship. In addition to direct financial support, there are the benefits of increased creativity and productivity in encouraging technology transfer which leads to the further promotion of economic growth and thus better public health.[17] Although the benefits are certain, one must question against what price this financial support is leveraged.

Are the gains made in the domain of public health – through technology, productivity, and creativity as supported by industry – great enough to counter the fact that prevention and nutrition do not receive support and are in fact discouraged?

Studies examining AIR have revealed that approximately 25% of investigators have industry relationships. Approximately two-thirds of academic institutions perform research for which they receive funding from start-ups that they hold equity in. The results of eight different studies aggregated show a significant relationship between industry sponsorship and pro-industry conclusions. There are also implications regarding the restriction of publication and data sharing.[18,19] This topic was explored in Chapter 3. When viewed in this light, AIR may affect the welfare of human subjects and could result in damage to the integrity and productivity of research, including the withholding of data and the tendency for research to pursue more commercial directions. Perhaps most importantly, these effects may result in the waning of public trust and support for academic research,[17] which, in conjunction with the recent state of federal funding and support for academic pursuits, is a dangerous prospect.

Following a discussion of the merits and dangers of AIR, students will discuss specifically how AIR affects health. This session will present an opportunity to discuss what the advantages and disadvantages of the preceding discussion mean, not in terms of industry but in terms of individual and community health. During this discussion, alternative relationships between money and health can be presented. Health insurance, medical malpractice insurance, and prescription drug costs, as well as the relationship between income and poor nutrition, are all important issues to be considered against the impact of money on health. Students will be asked to share stories of their experiences where finance affected a health outcome in a profound way.

Commercialism and nature

The focus of this session will be the possibility of limiting harmful practices while expanding and supporting mutually beneficial opportunities for industry and medicine to make money through initiatives that support environmental and personal health.

We will discuss how businesses promote health or damage it. Here we will introduce examples of the effects of business on the environment; industries discussed will include mining and agribusiness. We will consider pollution and efforts to promote environmental health. The recommended reading looks at the case of DuPont; its $3 billion a year petrochemicals division has endured a reputation as America's worst polluter.[20] In order to achieve sustainable growth DuPont is exploring the use of renewable resources like soy rather than expendable petroleum resources.

An example that illustrates the difficult nature of corporate social responsibility is McDonalds. That company has reduced waste by 300 million pounds per year since the 1980s and has become a major consumer of recycled materials. In addition, it has stopped using poultry treated with fluoroquinolones, an antibiotic that compromises the effectiveness of some antibiotics to treat humans. Sustainable fishing practices are supported by the company, as is the use of refrigerants that do not contain Freon and hydrofluorocarbons. In Sweden, the company uses only renewable sources of energy and serves organic food with a "happy meal" that includes vegetable nuggets and carrots.[20] Even with all these attempts at incorporating socially and environmentally responsible practices, the products marketed and sold, however they may be produced, are themselves questionable in terms of nutritional value.

Medicine's obligation to the environment

Private interests influence and support questionable practices, but, at the same time, medicine in many ways supports similarly questionable activities in industry. Physicians regularly prescribe pharmaceuticals produced through methods that degrade our environment and utilize certain treatment options for which devices or compounds leave few environmentally responsible disposal options. There are, on the other hand, many instances in which industry and medicine ally to generate revenue through health-promoting practices. For example, the Alder Group, a Canadian consulting firm, focuses on enabling businesses to "strengthen the capacity of organizations to make a positive impact on health."

In one session we seek to address whether or not medicine should place greater value on protecting the natural environment. We will present a broad summary of science's attitudes towards nature. Genetic reductionist approaches will be reviewed and ecological frameworks for a conservation approach to medicine will be considered against current paradigms. Existing conservation and environmental medicine approaches will be highlighted for students' consideration.

The conversation starter during this session will ask: Should medicine place greater value in nature? Do doctors have a professional obligation to advocate for a healthy environment? We will consider the links between illness and ecosystem impact, such as toxic emissions, land clearing, and climate change. Are current policies sufficient to address this growing area of concern? Prevention is in many respects dependent on the environmental variables we are exposed to. If medicine is to achieve a truly preventive stance, then surely the detrimental effects of the environment on our health should be of concern to medical practice. Conservation medicine and environmental medicine will be introduced here. Both of these disciplines strive to balance individual healing with global/environmental healing. It is through an introduction to these two disciplines that we hope students will adopt the notion that healing is a universal concept which, if confined to an individual's physiology and without regard to their environment, loses its meaning. If medicine chooses prevention as a basic tenet, it must also take responsibility for the industries and corporations it supports, their practices, and whether or not the support of such groups or entities aids or inhibits the concept of prevention. Just as we contemplated the corporate/industrial responsibility towards nature, here we contemplate medicine as an industry and ponder how socially responsible its practices are and should be. Students will be asked to discuss medicine's current value stance towards nature.

Professionalism in organizations

In our final session, we aim to return to our discussion of professionalism, reflecting on the various topics covered throughout the course. By this point students should begin to realize the breadth of the medical professional's role and various responsibilities. Typically, physicians are considered individuals who help other individuals.

The focus here is on the fact that physicians are representatives of healthcare institutions responsible for the health of entire communities. We will consider the impact that individual physicians can have on their organizations and, in turn, on the communities that they serve. As examples, the achievements of physicians actively engaged in social justice issues and green clinics will be examined.

The question at the heart of this session, which will be presented during the conversation starter, is: What roles and responsibilities do physicians have in organizational life and towards communities rather than individual patients? This discussion will lead to the creation of "ideal" mission statements for medical–professional organizations. Students will be asked to share attributes of ideal mission statements and then create one on their own.

Conclusion

There is a tendency to consider genetic advances and other molecular technologies as the future of medicine. The promises of personalized medicine are seen through an optimistic belief in technology but without fully considering the possibility of devastating depersonalization that may result from it. Today, some enjoy longer lives than years past, but these added years come at an ever-increasing price – financially, environmentally, and spiritually. The physicians of tomorrow will be practicing in a very different world in which the alterations in patterns of disease and the demographics of patient populations will offer major challenges. With prolonged lives resulting in larger aging populations, the prevalence of chronic diseases, like Alzheimer's and other dementias, will continue to increase, and, in addition, it is likely that infectious diseases, environmental toxic chemicals, and shortages of natural resources will contribute a greater share of suffering. The growing number of older people will be at risk for these threats to health as well as the impact of age-related chronic diseases. Children will be increasingly vulnerable to intergenerational equities. Healthcare resources will be more strained as the proportion of the population working that supports those resources decreases, and the number of those eligible to receive coverage increases. These economic limitations may contribute to greater political and social unrest, potentially contributing to greater global hostility that, in turn, may magnify ecological damage and health-related suffering.

The practice of medicine has become more complicated, and with it we have changing expectations of its practitioners. We now charge our healers with the duty of maintaining constant vigilance over the improvement of health at large. In addition, the forces at work against our health, such as poor nutrition and harmful environmental practices, are demanding attention. Healers of the future will increasingly be held accountable for addressing the detrimental health effects associated with these health behaviors and environmental toxic exposures.

If we are to see these expectations met, a new standard of medical education and a new social contract are necessary. Through this new social contract, we seek to empower patients with the responsibility for their own health. This new standard must introduce physicians to professionalism as we define it today, including strategies to quell the cynicism many medical students develop during their education, foster a global compassion and a spirit of environmental protection and healing, focus attention on prevention and nutrition, and forge ethical responsibility to uphold these values free from adulteration through the influence of industry.

Medical advances over the past century have been dramatic. Yet it is often unclear whether the costs associated with the introduction of new drugs, and technology, are justified by their impact on clinical care. These concerns have taken us away from the individualized care of the generalist family physician who had an in-depth knowledge of the lifestyles of their patients. Through technology, we may have removed some of the human touch from medicine. We are now in a position to reform the practice of medicine by reevaluating the education of physicians. We should pursue a grand vision of a healthier humanity, not solely through advances in technology but rather through our choice to respect ourselves, each other, and our natural world.

Acknowledgements

Preparation of this manuscript was supported by grant AG17511–03 Medical Goals in Dementia: Ethics & Quality of Life from the National Institutes of Health/NIA; and a grant from the Shigeo & Megumi Takayama Foundation, Tokyo, Japan.

References

1 Horowitz R (2004) *A Proposal for Radical Reform of Medical Education* (lecture to Faculty). Case School of Medicine and Health, Cleveland, OH.
2 Ludmerer KM (1999) *Time to Heal*. Oxford University Press, New York, NY.
3 Beck AH (2004) The Flexner Report and the standardization of American medical education. *JAMA*. **291**: 2139–40.
4 Flexner AA (1910) *Medical Education in the United States and Canada*. Carnegie Foundation for the Advancement of Teaching, New York, NY.
5 Academe (1999) Medical schools in the era of managed care: an interview with Arnold Relman. *Academe*. **85**: 16–23.
6 Morrill AC and Chinn CD (2004) The obesity epidemic in the United States. *J Public Health Policy*. **25**: 353–66.
7 Deen D (2004) Metabolic syndrome: time for action. *Am Fam Physician*. **69**: 2875–82.
8 Levitsky DA and Youn T (2004) The more food young adults are served, the more they overeat. *J Nutr*. **134**: 2546–9.
9 Prince JR (2004) Why all the fuss about portion size? Designing the new American plate. *Nutr Today*. **39**: 59–64.
10 Oh K, Hu FB, Cho E *et al.* (2005) Carbohydrate intake, glycemic index, glycemic load, and dietary fiber in relation to risk of stroke in women. *Am J Epidemiol*. **161**: 161–9.
11 Hayne CL, Moran PA and Ford MM (2004) Regulating environments to reduce obesity. *J Public Health Policy*. **25**: 391–407.
12 Epstein LH, Paluch RA, Consalvi A *et al.* (2000) Effects of manipulating sedentary behavior on physical activity and food intake. *J Pediatr*. **140**: 334–9.
13 UPENN (2000) UPENN School of Medicine Nutrition and Prevention Program. Available from www.med.upenn.edu/nutrimed/ (accessed April 15, 2005).
14 Reynolds P (1994) Reaffirming professionalism through the education community. *Ann Intern Med*. **120**: 609–14.
15 (1961) *Webster's Third New International Dictionary of the English Language*. Merriam-Webster Inc., Springfield, MA.
16 American Association for the Advancement of Science (1999) How to fund science: the future of medical research. Summary of plenary and breakout sessions. In: MO Hatfield, LE

Rosenberg and AH Teich (eds) *How To Fund Science: the future of medical research*. American Association for the Advancement of Science, Washington, DC.

17 Blumenthal D (1996) Ethics issues in academic–industry relationships in the life sciences: the continuing debate. *Acad Med.* **71**: 1291–6.

18 Frankel MS (1996) Perception, reality, and the political context of conflict of interest in university–industry relationships. *Acad Med.* 71: 1297–304.

19 Bekelman JE, Li Y and Gross CP (2003) Scope and impact of financial conflicts of interest in biomedical research: a systematic review. *JAMA.* **289**: 454–65.

20 Gunther M (2003) Tree huggers, soy lovers, and profits. *Fortune.* **147**: 98–100, 102, 104.

A proposed new grand strategy: an integrated health system for the 21st century

Norman J. Temple and Andrew Thompson

> *The reasonable man adapts himself to the world; the unreasonable one persists in trying to adapt the world to himself. Therefore all progress depends on the unreasonable man. (George Bernard Shaw in Reason)*

The problem

This book has presented a large body of evidence documenting that medicine, using the term in its widest sense, suffers from a colossal lack of fiscal control. In many cases the money simply flows straight down the drain in the form of unnecessary and overpriced expenditures. We have paid most attention to the situation in the USA, and that country is certainly the epicenter of the crisis, but there is no doubt that the problem is also serious in all other Western countries.

Chapters 3–8 catalogued the criminal level of waste that pervades all aspects of the pharmaceutical industry, starting at research, proceeding through clinical trials, thence on to the publishing of the findings, government approval of drugs for clinical use, development of a pricing and marketing strategy by the drug companies, and finally in the prescribing habits of doctors. Like an onion, as you peel back the layers, the smell gets worse, and you want to cry more. Quite apart from cost, a rational reorganization of the entire pharmaceutical enterprise would almost certainly result in many health gains for users of drugs, especially by the avoidance of drugs in situations where they are likely to do more harm than good. An excellent example of excessive spending is the use of high-priced medications for treating hypertension when, for most patients, other drugs, costing a fraction of the price, are just as effective and may even be safer. It is extremely difficult to quantify the extent of the financial wastage but there seems little doubt that drug costs could be cut by at least one-third without harming a single patient. Now as drug costs constitute almost 13% of total healthcare expenditures in the USA (2002 estimates),[1] this indicates that reform of the drug industry could shave around 4% to 5%, perhaps more, from total medical expenditures.

In Chapter 9 Temple and Fraser furnished evidence from the USA that medical expenditures could be cut by 20% to 30% simply by eliminating unnecessary medical interventions, such as much of the testing and consultations with specialists that serves no good purpose. And it is unlikely that this would result in any patient being denied a beneficial medical procedure. The strongest supporting evidence comes from comparisons of high-spending geographical areas with low-spending ones. Adding together the above two figures (4% to 5% plus 20% to 30%) we arrive at a total waste of 24% to 35%. These numbers may be compared with the analysis made by Sager and Socolar,[2] who estimated that about half of healthcare spending in the USA is eaten up by waste, excessive prices, and fraud (this was referred to in Chapter 9).

The above cases refer to wasteful spending in its purest form. Earlier chapters have also documented the large amount of excessive expenditure on medical interventions which, although mostly beneficial to health, are difficult to justify on the basis of cost. By this we mean that the cost, expressed as dollars per quality-adjusted life year (QALY), exceeds the amount that a society can reasonably afford if money were spent prudently. The case of statins exemplifies this problem: in Chapter 8 Temple and Thompson argued that there is strong evidence of huge overprescribing of this drug and consequent excessive spending. In chapters 11–14 we explored the area of screening for cancer, and here also we see much evidence that the cost is excessive for the benefits generated; this applies to cancer of the breast, cervix, and prostate.

Curing the problem

In this final chapter we make some proposals for reform of the medical enterprise, with a strong focus on reigning in wasteful and extravagant medical expenditures. We suggest how a Rolls Royce medicine can be traded in for a perfectly adequate VW medicine. However, we make no claim to being experts in the nitty-gritty of health policy management. Rather, our proposals are made as generic suggestions that should be applicable in a variety of countries.

Reigning in the cost of medicine is a matter of great urgency and importance. Medicine does not exist in splendid isolation from the rest of society's problems. The bill for the huge and ever-increasing costs of medicine is only paid by denying money to high-priority areas, such as environmental protection, education, and care for the less fortunate, both at home and around the world. It is no exaggeration to say that wasting billions on medical treatment is a crime when the inevitable consequence is cutbacks in essential but underfunded budgets.

Before these various changes to the practice of medicine can meet with any real success, there is a vital need for public education to explain why they are necessary.

A new approach to drug development

At the heart of the problem with drugs is profiteering and conflict of interest. If the experts involved at each step were motivated only by doing what is right, rather than what is best for their careers or their personal finances, then most of the problems we have discussed would spontaneously disappear. Clinical trials of drugs would be designed so that the results would be likely to demonstrate the true worth of the drug, or lack thereof. The results would be published, irrespective of how unwelcome they are to vested interests. Drug trials would be reviewed in an unbiased way, not by someone paid to draw the "right" conclusion.

The essential requirement is an independent agency responsible for conducting clinical trials of drugs. Pharmaceutical companies would submit proposals to this agency, including the evidence they have accumulated on the efficacy of the drug. A clinical trial would only be commenced if this were justified based on a full examination of the evidence, with careful consideration given to whether the new drug is apparently superior to existing drugs (or other treatments) and its likely cost-effectiveness.

When the proposed agency conducts clinical trials, it should adhere to the following principles:

- Clinical trials should be registered.
- The experimental drug should be compared with a standard drug or other treatment, if one exists, and not a placebo.
- Results should be published in a way that is clear and honest, warts and all.
- Findings must allow the reader to evaluate the real value of the drug; this means showing absolute risk reduction (not only relative risk) and number needed to treat for one patient to benefit (NNT).
- Where feasible and relevant, the effect of the drug on all-cause mortality should be shown.
- A realistic cost-analysis of the drug should be estimated, with findings shown in terms of QALYs.
- Postmarketing surveillance would be efficiently conducted and drugs would be withdrawn as soon as experts determined that this was in the public interest.

Writing review papers and clinical guidelines should only be done by experts who are free of conflict of interest.

Making a "wish list" of areas for reform is the easy part. The difficult bit, of course, is implementing them. It is highly predictable that the pharmaceutical industry will vigorously oppose all the required reforms. After all, turkeys don't vote for Christmas. Reform will only come when governments wake up to the crisis, recognize its true nature, and become resolved to impose a solution.

However, there have been some encouraging developments in recent years. In particular, two major steps have been taken to tackle the problem of nonpublication of studies that commercial interests, usually pharmaceutical companies, see as damaging to the profitability of their products. Eleven prominent medical journals issued a statement in 2001 that they would no longer publish the results of clinical trials where there was a contract that gave the sponsor the power to block publication.[3] Then, in 2004, the editors of the same medical journals went one step further. They implemented a policy, which came into effect in 2005, that they would only consider a clinical trial for publication if the trial were first registered on a register of trials.[4] The register must be accessible to the public at no charge. They stated in this declaration that: "Registration is only part of the means to an end; that end is full transparency with respect to performance and reporting of clinical trials." However, this still leaves a huge number of journals that have apparently not embraced these necessary changes in their editorial policies.

Pricing and marketing drugs

Even if all the above proposals were fully implemented, the pharmaceutical industry would still have ample opportunity to engage in excessive profiteering.

One way they have done that is in their pricing policies, as described in Chapter 6. The problems described apply mainly to the USA. Other countries, such as Canada, have developed systems that avoid many of these problems (which is why many Americans buy their drugs in Canada).

Much of the problem occurs at the interface between the pharmaceutical industry and doctors. As detailed in Chapter 5, drug companies have perfected their techniques to persuade doctors that a high-priced drug should always be used, even when a cheaper one is available. Adverts in medical journals reinforce the message. The result of this was graphically shown in Chapter 7 which documented the enormous sums of money that could be saved in Canada if doctors prescribed economically priced drugs, especially generics, rather than brand-name drugs, often given inappropriately. In Chapter 8 we focused on statins, and documented how, if current guidelines were implemented, there would be a huge increase in the level of extravagant spending.

Serious reforms need to be made to help solve this problem. First, drug company reps should be banned from talking to doctors: the entire system is so corrupt that it should be abolished. Instead, systems need to be developed so that doctors are given accurate and unbiased information to guide them in their prescribing. This could be done by way of medical journals (or other printed materials) combined with continuing medical education (CME).

Systems need to be introduced so that the organization that pays the drug bill refuses to pay an excessive amount. This requires action at the level of both drug prices and individual prescriptions. Drug prices can be set at the national level. In Canada the Patented Medicine Prices Review Board (PMPRB) has achieved some success in controlling the price of drugs. It has authority to limit the introductory price for new patented drugs and prevent prices for existing drugs from rising faster than the rate of inflation. For individual prescriptions, the key challenge is to avoid high-price patented drugs being sold when perfectly adequate low-priced generic drugs are available. Chapter 15 described one means to achieve this, namely the Reference Drug Program (RDP) in British Columbia, Canada. In the USA 39 states have already implemented mandatory generic substitution policies for Medicaid recipients.[5]

Evaluation of new medical findings

The above pertains specifically to drug development. But much of this is also relevant to other aspects of the development of new medical procedures and their evaluation. Medicine has a long history of adopting procedures which have not been properly evaluated. The emergence of "evidence-based medicine" in recent years is an implicit acknowledgment of this problem. Therefore, during the development of new medical interventions there is a need for careful evaluation by experts who are free of conflict of interest and can make an unbiased study. This should include a cost evaluation. If it appears that the likely cost of a proposed new procedure exceeds reasonable limits (which are discussed below), then further development is no longer justified. And if the procedure is already in use, then its further use should be terminated.

As an example of the need for this type of research, long-term trials are required that test whether each of the different types of screening procedures for cancer are truly effective. Such trials should carefully determine the cost-effectiveness of each intervention.

Cost limits, cost-effectiveness, and medicine

An essential component of a complete solution to the problem of overspending is to set cost limits on medical expenditures, a topic discussed in Chapter 1. These costs need to be expressed as cost (dollars) per QALY so that comparisons between diverse medical procedures can be objectively made. Our proposed medium-term goal is $50 000 per QALY, while $27 000 per QALY should be seen as both an ideal limit and a longer-term goal (in 2004 US dollars). We again emphasize that both these figures are very rough estimates and open to debate.

But before any real attempt can be made to impose cost limits, there is a need for an analysis of the cost of medical interventions. The procedure used is known as cost-effectiveness analysis (CEA). It has been actively researched and developed over many years.[6] Despite being heavy with imprecision and value judgments, CEA remains an invaluable tool. For example, if healthcare administrators have to consider various forms of intervention, say treating heart patients with drugs, surgery, or lifestyle education, then CEA can help them decide how to squeeze maximum value from a limited budget.

The best-known example of an attempt to incorporate CEA into medical decision-making took place in Oregon.[6] Known as the Oregon Health Plan, it was introduced in that state in 1994. The aim was to explicitly approve or deny medical services based on their cost. The plan did not end up actually saving any money. However, that was not due to intrinsic flaws in the use of imposed spending limits but to other factors related to the structure of the American healthcare system, such as increased numbers of people becoming eligible to receive health insurance.

No other state has attempted to emulate Oregon. Neumann[6] sees major cultural and political barriers in the USA that prevent that country from using CEA as an integral part of health policy so as to deny medical interventions on the basis of cost. But refusing to take decisive action will, of course, do nothing for the spending crisis in American medicine.

From a practical point of view a reasonable conclusion might be that if this is the best that can be achieved in the foreseeable future in order to curb wasteful extravagance, then it is a positive step. However, taking a longer-term and more optimistic perspective, if the people of Oregon can accept the principle that cost limits are necessary, surely so too can the rest of the American people.

Fortunately, resistance to CEA – and the implication of spending restrictions – is much weaker in other countries. CEA has been used, to a greater or lesser extent, in various countries, including Australia, Canada, the UK, and other parts of Europe. Neumann[6] examined the experiences of these countries and concluded that:

> ... CEA requires political will from politicians and policy makers ... [these experiences] prove that, given the right political circumstances, public officials can apply cost-effectiveness analysis openly. They confirm that the United State's failure to use CEA is driven more by its own cultural conditions than by the technique's inherent methodological shortcomings.

In order to be successful, cost limits must be applied rationally and in a way that does not alienate the public. We can point to two countries for inspiration as to how this can be done. In Australia the Pharmaceutical Benefits Advisory Committee (PBAC) advises the government as to which drugs should be included in the list of drugs which are subsidized by the government. CEA is a major criterion. While there is no hard and fast rule, drugs that cost in excess of $50 000 per QALY are unlikely to be accepted.[7] The UK has established the National Institute for Health and Clinical Excellence (NICE), which examines the value of both drugs and medical devices in terms of both clinical effectiveness and cost effectiveness. This agency is independent of government and releases reports that, with few exceptions, contain full details of its decisions. As in Australia there is no firm cost limit but drugs or devices costing above about $31 000 to $46 000 per QALY are likely to be rejected.[7,8]

The methodology for CEA is very much a "work in progress;" there are several critical issues that require further investigation. CEA is based on averages of many individuals, but no one individual corresponds to the average: one man's pain from migraine is quite different from that of the next man, and one woman's life expectancy gain from statins will be different from the next woman's. CEA is based on assumptions over how factors such as age, pain, and immobility affect quality of life. Is two years for a 30-year-old in full health equivalent to three years for an 80-year-old who has several infirmities? Another factor that should ideally be included in CEA modeling is nonmedical costs or gains. For example, a health promotion intervention in the workplace may include costs (such as hiring new personnel and purchase of exercise equipment) but also gains (such as reduced number of sick days).

In Chapter 1 we reviewed some of the sources of error in CEA and how these can easily lead to serious underestimations of the true cost of medical interventions. Commonly used CEA models are often seriously lacking in transparency and lend themselves to distortion. This results in wide ranges of estimates for the same basic procedure[9,10] and to unrealistically low costs. In Chapter 11 Luc Bonneux discussed CEA models used for screening of cancer and explained why they can generate misleading results; they typically overestimate the efficacy of the interventions and this results in screening appearing to be much more cost-effective than it really is.

Since current journal practice is to accept these cost analyses without requiring a detailing of all the assumptions and their effects, it can therefore be almost impossible to determine what exactly has been done and to critically evaluate the bottom line. In order to be credible CEA must be done in a transparent manner so that the assumptions made are clear. Such assumptions should include:

- The impact on health of the drug or intervention. (Was there an overoptimistic assumption as to the benefit of the drug? Was the estimate based on young patients but the drug will be given mainly to older patients? Were possible adverse effects factored in?)
- Future medicals costs avoided. (Did they include medical costs avoided in the next 10 years but ignore medical costs which will inevitably turn up at a later date?)
- Nonmedical costs. (Did they include such costs as administration?)

To facilitate this process and to lend credibility to CEAs, the study should be performed by an independent agency, not offered by the firms involved or others who stand to benefit from increased usage of the intervention being studied.

CEA needs to take a broad societal perspective. Medical and other interventions should be examined in order to determine their likely impact on public health. By this means it may be found that, for example, a modest reduction of air pollution in cities may be a more cost-effective means to improve health than a "breakthrough" drug that halves the death rate from an uncommon disease. Or, perhaps, that providing nutritious meals to children from low-income families does more to improve population health, in the long term, than screening for cancer of the cervix. We would then be able to make more intelligent decisions as to what interventions should be supported with public funding.

Schizophrenia in government policy

We now turn our attention to a huge obstacle to achieving rationality in medicine: government policy. In most countries it is governments that have control, direct or indirect, on spending related to the key components of medicine, including the use of CEA, spending limits, drug expenditure, and funding for medical research. In addition, governments control several of the key determinants of population health, such as tobacco taxes and food policy. The arguments made in this book make it essential, therefore, that governments should have a paradigm shift in their strategic approach to health and medicine. But often the actions of governments are contradictory, even schizophrenic.

The matter of agricultural subsidies illustrates this well. Governments in many Western countries appear to believe, that for reasons of economics, these are vitally important. This is done even when the consequence is that the subsidies alter food prices in such a way that people are encouraged to eat a less healthy diet. This has been well documented in Europe. There, the Common Agricultural Policy of the European Union gives subsidies to farmers and this brings about overproduction of various agricultural products. Issues of health are simply ignored in the decision-making process. For example, the subsidy on full-fat milk is 74% higher than that on skimmed milk, while large quantities of fruits and vegetables are withdrawn from the market and destroyed so as to maintain high prices.[11] Similarly, in both Europe and North America governments pay subsidies to tobacco farmers. But while these policies are being actively pursued by one section of government, simultaneously, other sections of the same governments advise people to eat a healthy diet (e.g. by promoting the American Food Pyramid) and not to smoke. One can easily point to many other cases of similar irrationality in government policies. For example, most governments have done nothing to compel food manufacturers to lower the salt content of food, despite the strong evidence that this will help counter hypertension at a negligible cost. Yet, at the same time, governments are willing to subsidize expensive medications for hypertension.

Clearly, there is a need for rationality and consistency in the areas of policies that relate to diet, lifestyle, health, and medicine. Governments need to develop a single integrated policy that embraces agricultural subsidies, taxation, health promotion, disease prevention, and medicine. Concrete ideas were discussed in Chapter 16 with regard to prices and subsidies on food and other commodities, as well as for legislation and policies controlling advertising and food labels. Policies in these areas should include a real cost-analysis so that, for example, the cost of subsidies for farmers producing tobacco and fat-rich milk are carefully assessed, taking into account not only their economic effects but also their impact on population health. Progress in giving these health issues their rightful place on the policy agenda has been painfully slow.

The practice of medicine and medical education

Solutions for many of the problems identified in this book will require changes in the way that doctors carry out their work. They will need to adopt an attitude of cost-effectiveness. The prescribing of drugs is certainly one area where doctors could quickly make a significant reduction in spending. Doctors would be greatly helped in this if they were given accurate information by unbiased experts rather than distorted information whose primary purpose is to boost profits for pharmaceutical companies. In other areas, such as referrals to specialists and advising patients on screening for cancer, there is again a critical need for doctors to receive proper guidance from experts who incorporate CEA into their overall judgments.

There are important barriers to be overcome before these changes can be made. One such barrier is the mindset that doctors develop during their medical training. Doctors typically see their only job as being to provide the best possible medical service to their patients. While commendable in many ways, this is, alas, a recipe for extravagance. Accordingly, significant changes are required in medical education so that doctors are schooled in the application of cost-effectiveness and spending limits.

At the same time doctors will need to practice health promotion in their work. At present this seldom goes much beyond encouraging people to quit smoking. The medical establishment must be persuaded that building fences at the top of the cliff makes much more sense than parking ambulances at the bottom. Here, we will briefly look at what are arguably the most critically important changes to medical practice. Doctors will need to develop their skills in this area, such as learning the most effective techniques for persuading their patients to eat more healthily and take more exercise. At present doctors receive little training in this. For example, one of us[12] has reported that Canadian doctors have serious deficiencies in their knowledge of nutrition. Here again, therefore, changes are required in the way that doctors are trained. Chapter 17 described a new course being used in medical education. More such highly innovative courses need to be developed. In addition, there is a need for more research into improved techniques by which doctors can carry out health promotion. The clear need for this was shown by the limited degree of success that has typically been seen when doctors have attempted to advise their patients to adopt a healthier lifestyle. This was briefly reviewed in Chapter 16.

It may well be that too many barriers prevent doctors from becoming effective practitioners of health promotion. If so, then doctors should refer patients to experts with the required skills, such as dietitians. Perhaps what is really needed is a whole new class of healthcare practitioners who specialize in health promotion. Such people would dispense advice across the whole lifestyle spectrum, including nutrition, exercise, smoking cessation, and behavior modification.

Conclusion

As the century unfolds people may look back with incredulity on today's world where narrow commercial interests and government laissez-faire predominate while the national health founders.

Modern medicine, most especially American medicine, suffers from the terrible disease of boundless self-confidence. What cannot be accomplished today will surely be achievable tomorrow, thanks to fantastic new breakthroughs that are just over the horizon: new drugs, more sophisticated computer-controlled gadgetry, genomic medicine, and so forth. They delude themselves into believing that there is no problem that another gazillion dollars cannot fix. But where will that gazillion dollars come from? Are people really prepared to make all those sacrifices to the environment, to education, to the protection of the needy that rapid cost escalation in medicine demands?

There is a story that in World War II the US Pacific fleet was steaming toward the enemy when they picked up an object on their radar. They repeatedly ordered it to get out of the way but to no avail. Finally, the reply came back: "We're a lighthouse." Medicine, also, needs to chart a new course.

References

1 Canadian Institute for Health Information (2005) *Drug Expenditure in Canada: 1985–2004*. Canadian Institute for Health Information, Ottowa.

2 Sagar A and Socolar D (2005) *Health Costs Absorb One-quarter of Economic Growth, 2000–2005*. Health Reform Program, School of Public Health, Boston University, Boston, MA. Available from http://dcc2.bumc.bu.edu/hs/ushealthreform.htm (accessed November 6, 2005).

3 Davidoff F, DeAngelis CD, Drazen JM *et al*. (2001) Sponsorship, authorship, and accountability. *Ann Intern Med*. **135**: 463–6.

4 DeAngelis C, Drazen JM, Frizelle FA *et al*. (2004) Clinical trial registration: a statement from the International Committee of Medical Journal Editors. *Ann Intern Med*. **141**: 477–8.

5 Centers for Medicare & Medicaid Services (2004) *Best Practices Among State Medicaid Drug Programs*. September. Available from www.cms.hhs.gov/medicaid/drugs/strategies.pdf (accessed November 13, 2005).

6 Neumann PJ (2005) *Using Cost-effectiveness Analysis to Improve Health Care*. Oxford University Press, Oxford.

7 Henry DA, Hill SR and Harris A (2005) Drug prices and value for money. The Australian Pharmaceutical Benefits Scheme. *JAMA*. **294**: 2630–2.

8 Pearson SD and Rawlins MD (2005) Quality, innovation, and value for money. NICE and the British National Health Service. *JAMA*. **294**: 2618–22.

9 Jefferson T and Demicheli V (2002) Quality of economic evaluation in health care. *BMJ*. **324**: 313–4.

10 Pignone M, Saha S, Hoerger T, Lohr KN, Teutsch S and Mandelblatt J. Challenges in systematic reviews of economic analyses. *Ann Intern Med*. **142**: 1073–9.

11 Elinder LS (2004) The EU Common Agricultural Policy from a health perspective. *Eurohealth*. **10**: 13–16.

12 Temple NJ (1999) Survey of nutrition knowledge of Canadian physicians. *J Am Coll Nutr*. **18**: 26–9.

Index

Abraham, J 38
Abramson, John 56, 57, 97
absolute risk reduction 15–16
academic–industry relationships
    (AIRs) 13–14, 22–8, 31–3, 171–2
  setting up private companies 13–14
  see also conflicts of interest (COIs);
    doctor–industry interactions
ACE inhibitors 143, 145
Action Heart (England) 155, 157
Adair, RF 56
Adalat XL.® (nifedipine) *83*, 84
adverse drug reactions
  failure to report 24
  postapproval risks 44
  postmarketing surveillance 44–5
advertisements
  direct-to-consumer 41, 47–8, 58–9
  industry spending patterns 57–8
  in journals 30–1, 57–8, 59
  for junk food 159, 160
  misleading statements 15–16
  regulation mechanisms 47–9
  return on investment rates 59
AIRs *see* academic–industry relationships
Alder Group 173
all-cause mortality measures 16, 94
ALLHAT study (2002) 87
Altace® (ramipril) 84
Angell, M 21–2, 24–5, 27, 54
angina treatments *83*, 84, 143, 145
angiotensin-converting enzymes (ACE) 84
animal studies 10
antibiotic prescribing 104–5
antidepressants 20–1, 86
  brand vs. generic drugs *83*, 86
  cost savings *83*
  drug regulation issues 38–9, 40
  use with children 40
Apotex 29
arthritis treatments
  brand vs. generic drugs *83*, 85, 87–8
  clinical research issues 24
  cost containment measures 143
  cost savings *83*
  development and marketing
    concerns 23, 40, 41, 43, 46, 87–8

drug regulation concerns 23, 40, 41, 43,
  46
aspirin 97, 99
Association of the British Pharmaceutical
  Industry (ABPI) 49
asthma research 24–5
AstraZeneca 29, 59
ATP III guidelines 97
Australia, drug regulation agencies 42–3
avian flu, drug pricing tactics 63–4

Baker, GR *et al.* 106
Bannerman, G *et al.* 106
Baume Report 43
Baum, Michael 127
Bayer 64–5
Bayh-Dole Act 32
BC Pharmacare
  aims and rationale 139
  background and history 139–41
Bekelman, JE *et al.* 28
benzodiazepines, drug regulation issues 38
Bero, LA and Rennie, D 21, 25
Bhandari, M *et al.* 27
biases in cancer screening 115
  in publications 115–16
biases in clinical trials 11–12, 20
  in selection of patients 24–5
  in study design 27
  see also conflicts of interests (COIs)
bird flu, drug pricing tactics 63–4
Blumenthal, D *et al.* 29, 30
Bodenheimer, T 25, 30, 32
Bolaria, SB and Dickenson, HD 27
Bonneux, Luc 17, 96–7, 98, 126
Boots Pharmaceuticals 29
bowel cancer screening 119
brand loyalty 55, 75
breast cancer screening 125–6
  adverse effects 127–8
  costs involved 128–9
  effectiveness concerns 112–18, 126–7
  studies 17, 121–3, 125
  study reviews 126–7
"Bristol-Myers Squibb" lawsuit 29
British Medical Journal, analysis of
  advertisements 57–8

Business Transformation Strategy
(Canada) 42

calcium channel blockers (CCBs) *83*, 84,
144
Campbell, EG *et al.* 23, 33
Canada
cost containment initiatives 88,139–49
drug regulation agencies 37–8, 42, 46,
48–9
drug spending patterns 53, 140–1
funding for research 22–3
healthcare expenditure 1
policy on use of placebos 12, 27
regulation of drug promotion 48–9
studies on breast screening 121–3, 125
threats to price controls 88
Canadian Coordinating Office on Health
Technology Assessment
(CCOHTA) 29
Canadian Medical Association Journal 57
cancer
life extension calculations 16–17
preventative measures 153
tumour growth patterns 113–14
see also screening for cancer
CanWest News Service 23–4
Case Western Reserve University
(Ohio) 167–74
CEA (cost-effectiveness analysis) 181–3
Celebrex® (celecoxib) 28–9, *83*, 85, 87–8
Center for Biologics Evaluation and
Research (CBER) 36
Center for Drug Evaluation and Research
(CDER) 36, 44
cervical cancer screening 119, 131–6
adverse effects 132–3
cost-effectiveness 134–5
efficacy 133
Chew, LD *et al.* 56
children
antibiotic use 104–5
antidepressant use 40
and drug safety concerns 40
cholesterol-lowering treatments
clinical guidelines 97, 98
generic vs. brands 82–4, *83*
lifestyle changes 93–4
and use of aspirin 97, 99
see also statins
Choudhry, NK *et al.* 30
Cipla (India) 64

Cipro® 64–5, *66*
"clientele pluralism" 37
clinical guidelines 80, 87–9, 98
clinical trials 10–19
academic–industry relationships
(AIRs) 13–14, 22–8, 31–3, 171–2
design concerns 27
error sources 13–14, 17–18
ethical considerations 12–13
expenditure on studies 24
ideal vs. real studies 21
key features 11
legal disputes 29
nonpublication and delayed
publication 29
other forms of research 9–13
presentation of results 94–6
publishing biases and errors 14–18,
27–31, 103
reforms needed 178–9
registration policies 179
reviews and meta-analysis 18, 30–1,
103, 180–1
translating into practice 18–19
use of endpoint measures 94
see also biases in clinical trials; conflicts of
interest (COIs)
CME *see* continuing medical education
(CME)
colorectal cancer screening 119
Common Agricultural Policy 183
Coney, S 48
conferences and symposia 56–7, 88
conflicts of interest (COIs) 20–33
in academic/medicine/commerce
partnerships 31–3, 171–2
in approval and funding stages 22–3
in drug regulation 45–9
in predictive genetic testing 111
in production of guidelines 87, 98, 801
in publication of findings 27–31
in review of publications 30–1
in risk disclosures 25–6
in study designs 27
in subject selection 23–5
see also biases in clinical trials
Conrad, P and Leiter, V 76
continuing medical education (CME)
involvement of industry 56–7, 87–8
on prescribing behaviors 87–9
contract research organizations (CROs) 23
Cooper, RJ and Schriger, DL 58

coronary heart disease treatments
  cost-effectiveness concerns 96–8
  lifestyle changes 93–4, 153
  prevention programmes 155–6
  use of aspirin 97, 99
cost analysis approaches 2–3, 112–13
cost containment 4–8
  aims and goals 8
  ethical determinants 5–7
  future directions 148–9
  government policies 4–5, 183–4
  international initiatives 139–40, 148,
    149
  programs and approaches 88–9, 139–49
  role of insurance industry 4
  target drug classes 143–5
  use of analysis tools 6–7, 181–3
cost of health promotion 162
cost of medical interventions
  background 1–2
  calculations and comparative analysis
    2–3, 112–13, 181–3
  doctor "awareness" 86–7
  imposing limits 4–7
cost recovery fees see user fees
cost-effectiveness models 2–3, 181–3
  see also cost of medical interventions
COX-2 inhibitors 83, 85, 87–8
  see also Vioxx® (rofecoxib)
Crestor® (rosuvastatin) 59, 82–4, 83

Danish Cochrane Center 116
Davis, P 106
DCIS (ductal cancer in situ) 127–8
Declaration of Helsinki 12
detailing 54–6
  return on investment rates 59
diabetes, drug regulation issues 40–1
dialysis 4
dietary control measures 93–4,167–9
direct-to-consumer advertising (DTCA) 41,
  47–8, 58–9
  industry expenditure patterns 58
disease prevention see prevention of disease
diuretics 83, 84
Division of Drug Marketing, Advertising,
  and Communication (DDMAC)
  47–8
DNA testing 110–11
doctor–industry interactions
  research/phase III trials 23–5, 27, 75
  role of sales representatives 54–6

use of conferences and medical
    education packages 56–7, 87–8
  use of free samples 55–6
  use of gifts 55–6
  use of rebates and financial
    inducements 74–5
doctors "as gatekeepers" 103–5
double blind trials 11–12
drug development
  costs involved 69–70, 140
  funding and approval 22–3
  influence of commerce 22–5, 27, 31–3,
    171–2
  and "me-too drugs" 53, 59, 72
  new approaches 178–9
  patent control mechanisms 63, 71, 74,
    88
  risk analysis and management 14–16,
    24, 25–6
  therapeutic values 72
  vs. use of generics 83, 86–9
  see also clinical trials
drug pricing see pricing of drugs
drug regulation see regulation of drugs
Drug Safety Oversight Board (US) 44
drug safety postmarketing see adverse drug
    reactions; postmarketing surveillance
drug spending
  average spend per person (USA) 102
  cf. total health expenditure
    (Canada) 140–1
  projected global sales 53
  see also healthcare expenditure
drug-related diseases 104
drug-related mortality 105–6
DuPont 172
DuVal, G 24, 32

Economist 123
Eddy, DE 133
Effexor XR® (venlafaxine) 86
elderly patients 102, 104
Eli Lily 21
environmental influences 172–3
epidemiological studies 9–10
ethical issues
  setting medical cost limits 4–8
  use of placebos 12–13, 27
  see also conflicts of interest (COIs);
    regulation of drugs
European Atherosclerosis Society 93

European Medicines Agency (EMEA)
44–5, 46
European Public Assessment Reports
(EPARs) 46
European Union (EU), postmarketing
surveillance 44–5
evidence-based medicine 180–1
exercise regimes 154, 160
expenditure on drugs *see* drug spending
Ezzati-Rice, TM *et al.* 102

false negatives 131
false positives 116
breast screening 128
cervical screening 131, 132–3
Family Heart Study (UK) 156
financial incentives 13
and patient recruitment 24–5
and university research 13–14
see also user fees
Fisher, ES *et al.* 105
"five-a-day" fruit and vegetable
campaign 154
Flexner, Abraham 166
fluoxetine *83*, 86
Food and Drug Administration (FDA) 12,
22, 36–7
effects of deregulation 39–41
funding and resources 39, 47
impact of user fees 39–41
openness and transparency 45–8
regulation of drug promotion 47–8
food and nutrition
government policies towards 158–61,
183
healthy eating campaigns 154–62
training for doctors 167–9
Food Politics (Nestle) 161
4S trial 95, *96*
Fraser Institute 146
Fraser, Joy 45
fraud 141
"free market pricing" 71
funding research 22–3
academia–industry affiliations 13–14,
27–8
and publication bias 27–31
see also user fees

generic drugs
cf. brand names *83*
cost savings *83*

and prescribing behaviors 86–9
for anthrax threats 64–5
for arthritis 85
for avian flu 63–4
for depression 86
for high cholesterol 82–4
for HIV/AIDS 65
for hypertension 84
for peptic ulcers/heartburn 85–6
"generic substitution" policies 141
genetic testing 110–11
German Cardiovascular Prevention
Study 155
gifts and inducements 55–6
Glassman, PA *et al.* 30
GlaxoSmithKline (GSK) 21, 65, 72
Gleevec® 68
Goodlee, Fiona 161
Goozner, M 71
Gøtzsche, PC 32–3
Gøtzsche, PC and Olsen, O 126–7
Gueriguian, Dr John 40
guidelines *see* prescribing guidelines

H_2-antagonists 143, 145
Hailey, D 29
Harmon, G and Val Sherwal, V 32
Hartley, H 76
Health Action International 23, 26
Health Canada 37
Health Insurance Plan of New York
(HIP) 122
health promotion *see* prevention of
disease
healthcare expenditure 102, 106
current levels 1, 53, 102
drivers 141
ethically set limits 1, 5–7
future projections 1, 53
and higher mortality rates 105–6
Healy, David 20–1
Heart Protection Study (HPS) 94, 95–6,
96
Henderson, JA and Smith, JJ 32
HIV vaccines 29
Holbrook, Anne 29
Horton, Richard 127
hydrochlorothiazide *83*, 84
hypertension treatments 59–60, *83*, 84, 87
cost containment measures 144, 145
generic vs. brands *83*, 84
review biases 30

iatrogenic diseases 104, 105–6, 114, 115
Immune Response Corporation 29
IMS Health survey 56
information for study participants 25–6
informed consent 12–13, 25–6
"innovative drugs" 71, 72
insurance industry 4
"intention to treat" 95
International Agency for Screening on
         Cancer (IARC) 123
International Convention on
         Harmonization of Good Clinical
         Practice 22
"interval cancers" 116

JAMA 105
James, WPT and Ralph, A 161
Jeffery, RW *et al.* 157
journal advertising 27–31, 57–8, 59, 103
    see also publishing research reports
junk food 154, 159–61
    advertising 159, 160
    government policies 159–60

Kahn, James 29
Kaiser Family Foundation 58, 106
"kickback" schemes 75
Kopparberg (Sweden) 115–16

laboratory studies 10
Lamm, Richard 7
Lancet 44, 59, 127
Lawson, GW 43
lead pollution 160
lead time 114
left-ventricular assist devices 4
legal disputes, suppressed publications 29
length time 114
Lewis, S *et al.* 29
Lexchin, J 38
Lexchin, J and Kawachi, I 48
Lexchin, J *et al.* 28
Lieberwitz, RL 32
life-years gained (LYGs) 2
lifestyle changes 81
    for cholesterol lowering 93–4
    community-based programmes 154–5
    impact of initiatives 157
    physician-initiated 156–7
    work-based campaigns 155–6
    see also prevention of disease
Light, DW and Lexchin, J 70

Light, DW and Warburton, RN 69–70
Linder, JA *et al.* 104
LIPID trial 94–5, *96*
Lipitor® (atorvastatin) 82–4, *83*
Lofgren, H and de Boer, R 42–3
Los Angeles Times 40
Losec® (omeprazole) *83*, 85–6
Love, J 30
Low Cost Alternative Program (LCA) 141
Ludmerer, Kenneth 166–7
Lumpkin, Dr Murray 40–1

McArthur, W 146
McDonalds 172–3
McGregor, M 144
Maclure, M *et al.* 142
Malmö Swedish screening trial 126
mammography (MA) *see* breast cancer
         screening
market creation strategies 76
market expansion strategies 75–6
Marketed Healthcare Products Regulatory
         Agency (MHRA) 40–1, 44–5
marketing activities
    control and regulation 47–9
    industry investment data 140
    role of CME packages 56–7
    use of direct-to-consumer
            advertising 41, 47–8, 58–9
    use of journal advertisements 27–31, 59
    see also sales tactics
Marshall, T 97
"maximum allowable cost" (MAC) 88
"me-too drugs" 53, 59, 72
Medawar, C and Hardon, A 38–9, 76
medical education and health
         promotion 166–75
    background and rationale 166–9
    curriculum planning 169–70
    curriculum topics 169–74
medical professionalism 170–1, 173–4
medicalization of conditions 76
Medicare 4
Medicines Act 1968 38
Medicines Commission 38–9
    see also Marketed Healthcare Products
            Regulatory Agency (MHRA)
Melander, H *et al.* 28
Merck 41, 46, 87
    see also Vioxx® (rofecoxib)
meta-analysis 18
    see also reviews of clinical trials

Mill, John Stuart 5
Minnesota Heart Health Program
    (Upper Midwest) 155
Mintzes, B et al. 58
Morin, K et al. 24
mortality from iatrogenic causes 105–6
mortality risk assessments 16–18
Mosholder, Dr Andrew 40–1
Muijrers, PEM et al. 56
Munro, M 24, 25–6
Murray, E et al. 58

naproxen 83, 85
National Cholesterol Education Program
    (NCEP) III guidelines 97, 98
Nature 30
NCEP guidelines see National Cholesterol
    Education Program (NCEP) III
    guidelines
Nemeroff, Charles 21
Nestle, Marion 161
net present value (NPV) calculations 68–9,
    68
New England Journal of Medicine 22, 31, 54
New York Times 64, 127, 129
New Zealand
    cost containment measures 139, 148, 149
    direct-to-consumer advertising 48
Nexium® (esomeprazole) 83, 85–6
NICE (National Institute for Health and
    Clinical Excellence) 182
nitrates 143, 145
NoFreeLunch website 68
non-pharmacological treatments see
    prevention of disease
nonsteroidal anti-inflammatory drugs
    (NSAIDs)
    brand vs. generic 83, 85
    commercial influence on prescribing
        guidelines 87–8
    cost containment measures 143
    cost savings 83
    development and marketing of Vioxx®
        23, 40, 41, 43, 46, 87–8
    research participant biases 25
Norvasc® (amlodipine) 83, 84
number needed to treat (NNT) 15, 95
Nurses' Health Study (US) 153
nutrition education, in medical
    curricula 167–9
Nyquist, AC et al. 104
Nyström group 115

obesity 154, 168
off-label uses 75–6
Olivieri, Nancy 29
Olsen, O and Gøtzsche, PC 126–7
omeprazole 83, 85–6
Oregon Health Plan 181
Oregon Health Resources Commission 85,
    89
Orlowski, JP and Wateska, L 57
Ostergötland breast cancer screening trials
    (Sweden) 115–16
"overall mortality" 16
OXCHECK study (UK) 156

PAAB see Pharmaceutical Advertising
    Advisory Board (Canada)
Pantaloc® (pantoprazole) 83, 85–6
Pap tests see cervical cancer screening
paroxetine 21, 38–9
participants see research participants
Patented Medicines Prices Review Board
    (PMPRB) (Canada) 88, 140, 146–7,
    180
patents 13, 74
    control mechanisms (Canada) 88
    effects on pricing 71
    extensions and protection tactics 71
    impact on innovation 63, 74
patient selection procedures see selection of
    research participants
patient volunteers see research participants
Pawtucket Heart Health Program (Rhode
    Island) 155
Paxil® (paroxetine) 21, 38–9
Perlis, CS et al. 28
Pfizer 21, 69, 88
Pharma Sales Force Effectiveness Congress
    (2005) 55
Pharmacare see BC Pharmacare
Pharmaceutical Advertising Advisory Board
    (PAAB) (Canada) 48–9
Pharmaceutical Benefits Advisory
    Committee (PBAC) (Australia) 182
pharmaceutical industry 101
    drug pricing strategies 63–78, 179–80
    influence on clinical trials 13–14, 22–8,
        31–3, 171–2
    influence on publishing bodies 27–31
    patent control mechanisms 63, 71, 74,
        88
    responsibility for excessive costs
        103

see also advertisements; marketing activities

Pharmacia 28–9

PharmaNet 141–2, 144

physician training *see* medical education

pilot studies 10

placebos 12–13, 27, 93–5

PMAC *see* Patented Medicines Prices Review Board (PMPRB) (Canada)

pollution 160, 172–3

postmarketing surveillance 44–5

pravastatin 84

"precautionary principle" 37

preliminary studies 10

prescribing behaviors 86–9, 103–5
  antibiotics 104–5
  introducing control measures 141–2, 145–6

"prescribing cascade" 104

prescribing guidelines 80–1, 87, 98

prescription costs 88, 102
  see also drug spending; pricing of drugs

Prescription Drug User Fee Act 1992 (PDUFA) 39

prevention of disease 80–1, 152–63
  challenges 153–4
  cost-effectiveness 161–2
  government policies 158–61
  health promotion campaigns 154–6
  impact of health promotion 157
  as medical intervention 156–7
  problems and barriers 160–1

"price controls" 71
  see also cost containment

pricing of drugs 63–78
  buyer's perspectives 76–8
  consumer protest schemes 77–8
  corporate decision-making models 67–9, 68
  influence of patents 71–2, 88
  international comparisons 65, 67, 88
  lifecycle models 68
  prescriber's behaviors 86–9
  production costs vs. mark-up prices 63–7
  R & D costs 69–70
  reforms and new directions 179–80
  restrictive practices and monopolies 74
  seller's perspectives 72–3
  seller's tactics 73–6
  see also cost containment; drug spending

"primary" analysis (cost of health effects) 112–13

principal-agent theory 43

Productivity Commission of Australia 63

professionalism in medicine 170–1, 173–4

prostrate cancer screening 119–20, 125–6

proton pump inhibitors *83*, 85–6

Prozac® 20–1, 28

"pseudodiagnosis" 114

psychological interventions 81

publishing research reports
  commercial influences 27–31, 103
  error sources 14–18, 27–31
  selective use of findings 28–9
  suppression of findings 29, 179

quality-adjusted life years (QUALYs) 2–3, 125, 181–2
  by health promotion 162
  by screening 125

Raffle, AE *et al.* 133, 134, 135

ramipril *see* Altace® (ramipril)

Ranbaxy 65

randomized controlled trials (RCTs)
  design concerns 27
  ethical considerations 12–13
  key features 11
  publication biases 27–31
  selection of patients 11, 23–5
  sources of error 13–14, 17–18
  use of placebos 12–13
  see also clinical trials; published research reports

"rebates" and financial incentives 74–5

reciprocity 56

recruiting volunteers *see* selection of research participants

Reference Drug Program (RDP) 88, 139–49
  aims and rationale 139–40
  key drug classes 143–4, 145
  background and history 139–41
  conflicts and opposition 145–7
  evaluation methods and studies 144, 147–8
  future concerns and directions 148–9

Reference Pricing 71, 88–9

regulation of drugs 36–50
  background and history 36–9
  commercial influences 22–3, 45–6
  deregulation effects 39–43
  introduction of user fees 39–43

openness and transparency 45–6
promotion and advertising controls 47–9
resubmissions 45
see also postmarketing surveillance
regulatory capture theory 43
"reimportation" 71
relative risk 14–16
Remune® 29
Rennie, D 29
research and development (R&D) costs 69–70
industry investment data 70, 140
research on drugs *see* clinical trials; drug development
research ethics *see* ethical issues
research participants
consent issues 25–6
selection concerns 11–12, 23–5
research regulation *see* regulation of drugs
researchers
financial incentives 13, 24–5
industry affiliations 27, 172
role conflicts 24–5
unethical behaviors 103
reviews of clinical trials 30–1, 103
new directions in evaluation 180–1
Rezulin® (troglitazone) 40–1
risk analysis
misleading statements 15–16
presentation methods 14–15
risk of death measures *see* mortality risk assessments
risk disclosure
consent concerns 25–6
controlling and preventing 29
Ritter, P 29
Roche 63–4
Rochon, P *et al.* 25
rofecoxib *see* Vioxx® (rofecoxib)
Roughead, EE *et al.* 89

Sackett, DL and Oxman, AD 33
Sager, A and Socolar, D 105
sales representatives 54–6
sales tactics
use of conferences and medical education packages 56–7
use of free samples 55–6
use of gifts 55–6
see also marketing activities
salt intake 161

samples of drugs 55–6
Schafer, A 28–9, 33
Schuppli, CA and MacDonald, M 25
Schwartz, B *et al.* 104
scientists *see* researchers
screening for cancer 112–20, 180–1
benefits vs. costs 123, 125–9
cost effectiveness analysis challenges 3, 112–13
data validity 115–16
detection of "interval cancers" 116
Dutch MISCAN economic model 116–17
effects on incidence and mortality 116–18, *117*, 123
efficacy studies 112–13, 116–18, 121–3, 126–7, 180–1
evaluation criteria 122–3
for breast cancer 112–18, 125–30
for cervical cancer 119, 131–6
for colorectal tumours 119
for prostrate tumours 119
fundamental principles 113–14
incidence of false positives 116, 132
litigation impacts 116
potential harmful effects 17–18, 115, 118–20, 127–8
problems attributing cause of death 114–15
promoter interests 123
Searle 88
"secondary analysis" (cost of health effects) 112–13
selection of research participants
conflicts of interest 23–5
general concerns 11–12, 45
use of placebos 12–13
selective serotonin reuptake inhibitors (SSRIs) 20–1
drug regulation issues 38–9, 40
use with children 40
selenium 153
self-care therapies 81
serotonin and norepinephrine reuptake inhibitors (SNRIs) *83*, 86
Seroxat® (paroxetine) 21, 38–9
Shearer, Frederick Mike 69
Shojania, Dr Kam 24
"slippery biases" 115
"smart regulation" 42
smoking 153, 154, 157, 158, 161

SNRIs *see* serotonin and norepinephrine reuptake inhibitors
Soumerai, SB *et al.* 88–9
sponsorships *see* funding research
SSRIs *see* selective serotonin reuptake inhibitors
Stagnitti, MN 102
Stanford Five-City Project (California) 155
Starfield, Barbara 105
statins 59, 93–9
    cost savings *83*
    cost-effectiveness 96–8
    generic vs. brand names 82–4, *83*
    key studies *96*
    marketing and advertising 59
    presentation of research findings 14–16, 94–6, *96*
    suppression of research findings 29
    validity of clinical trials 93–6, *96*
    vs. dietary control measures 93–4
Stelfox, HT *et al.* 30
"sticky bias" 115
subjects *see* research participants
sugar intake 161
symposia *see* conferences and symposia
Synthyroid 29

Tamiflu® 63–4
tax relief 31
terminal illnesses and clinical trials, consent issues 26
Therapeutic Goods Administration (TGA) 42–3
Therapeutic Products Directorate (TPD) 37–8, 42, 46
Therapeutics Initiative (TI) 142
tobacco industry 158, 161
"Tommy" Thompson 64–5
TPD *see* Therapeutic Products Directorate (TPD)
training and education *see* medical education
Treatwell Program (New England) 156
troglitazone *see* Rezulin® (troglitazone)

Troy, Daniel 48
Two County Trial (Sweden) 116

Uhegarty, K *et al.* 86
Under Reference Pricing 88
United Kingdom
    drug promotion regulation 49
    drug regulation agencies 38–9, 49
    lifestyles and health 154
    policies towards drug pricing 77
    policies towards R & D 77
United States
    drug pricing systems 63–7
    healthcare expenditure 1, 102, 106
    lifestyles and health 154
    public satisfaction with healthcare 106–7
university research
    influence of commerce 13–14, 31–3
    setting up private companies 13–14
UPENN medical education programs 168
US Preventative Services Task Force 113, 126
US Public Citizen 140
user fees 39–43

venlafaxine 86
Viagra® 68
Vioxx® (rofecoxib) 23, 40, 41, 43, 46, 87–8
volunteer subjects *see* research participants

Wall Street Journal, on AZT 65
Warner-Lambert 40–1
Washington Post 64
Watkins, C *et al.* 56
Wiktorowicz, ME 37
Wilcox, S *et al.* 156
Wolfe, S 102
Women's Health Action Trust (New Zealand) 48
Woolley, M and Propst, SM 106
work-based health promotion campaigns 155–6